A MANUAL ON HUMANICS

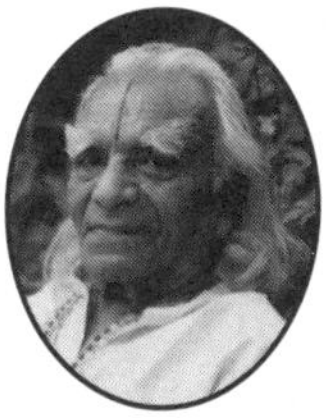

"I always tell people, live happily and die majestically"

—B.K.S. Iyengar

YOG TRADITION OF INDIA

Yog is a pride possession of our great Indian tradition. It is a science, a faculty, a philosophy, a religion and a culture. The science of Yog contains entire thought of man. Yog knowledge can offer the highest goal and bliss of life. An anthology of the discourses were expounded by Prashant Iyengar for the students, scholars and sadhakas of Yog at different points of time. The readers, while learning Mantra Yog, Laya Yog, Hatha Yog, Raja Yog, Kundalini Yog, Nada Yog, Nama Yog as kinds of Jnana Yog, Karma Yog, Bhakti Yog and Dhyana Yog can get acquainted with many facets of Yog, They will learn that Yog is a way of Life. It is the sadhna of life. The engaging style of narration will appeal to the readers' brain and heart while they imbibe the knowledge of Yog, For easy comprehension, the words in the Sandhis are separated in the Sanskrit quotations. The books written by Prasant S. Iyengar selected to be published under the series are:

1. **Ashtanga Yoga of Patanjali:** *Philosophy, Religion, Culture, Ethos and Practices*
2. **Discourses on Yog**
3. **Manual on Humanics**
4. **Pranayama:** *A classical and traditional approach*

PRASHANT S. IYENGAR

A MANUAL ON HUMANICS

New Age Books
New Delhi (India)

A MANUAL ON HUMANICS

ISBN: 978-81-7822-479-4

First NAB Edition: Delhi, **2016**

Published by
NEW AGE BOOKS
A-44 Naraina Industrial Area, Phase-I
New Delhi (India)-110 028
E-mail: nab@newagebooksindia.com
Website: www.newagebooksindia.com

NAB Cataloging-in-Publication Data
A MANUAL ON HUMANICS
ISBN 978-81-7822-479-4
(About the Series, Contents, Candid words from the heart, Tale of the title, Introduction)

Printed and published by
RP Jain for NAB Printing Unit
A-44, Naraina Industrial Area
Phase-I, New Delhi-110 028. India

TRADITION OF YOG

There are many traditions in classical yog and there is great scope for research. But all classical yog find trace in what the Mahabharata mentions:

हिरण्यगर्भो योगस्त वक्ता नान्यः पुरातनः।

Mahabharata later clarifies that the Hiranyagarbha is Paramatma Sriman Narayana who is the Sarva- Antaryami and He is the first speaker of yog. Hiranyagarbha Yog has been maintained in bits and pieces in Pancharatra. Ahirbudhnya Samhita mentions that He gave discourses on chitta-vritti nirodha kind of yog which has Abhyasa-Vairagya and Ishvara- Pranidhana as means. The schemes of Ashtanga Yog too find a mention here. This is the basis of Patanjali's Yog. This main stream of yog received many contributions. Apart from the Pancharatra originated Vaishnava Agamas, the other major contributions were from Tantras, Shaiva agamas and Shakta Agamas. Many of the yogic concepts of Kriya, Mudra and Bandha were given by Shaiva-Shakta agamas and Tantras. The North Indian tradition of yog was greatly influenced by these. So much so that Lord Shiva became the source of yog for them. Hatha-yogic tradition has strong base in Shaiva cult of yog. The Natha-Sampradaya puts Adinath (Shiva) as origin of yog. We have great texts such as Hatha yog pradipika, Gheranda samhita, Shiva samhita and prolific works ascribed to Gorakhnath.

Dattatreya who advised yog to Sankruti must also be considered here. This piece of instruction is preserved for us in the Shandilya Upanishad. Gheranda rishi in his samhita has the yog where he puts Pratyahara before Pranayama while usually all traditions maintain the Pranayama to Prattyahara process. This is quite a significant revolution.

The Bhagwad Gita revived the Karma yog tradition which Bhagwan Himself says was instructed earlier (in Vaikuntha) to Vivasvan (Surya). The Gita mentions the main forms of yoga which are

- **Jnana Yog**
- **Dhyana Yog**
- **Karma Yog**
- **Bhakti Yog**

There is great significance when Vyasa calls Gita as Brahma vidya, Upanishad and Yog shastra in the colophone of each chapter. Each chapter is called as a kind of yog and thus eighteen chapters give us eighteen yogs.

The Yogopanishads posit that Ashtanga Yog is fount-hole of all various yogs. Then there are different yogs in different levels. The first level is Ashtanga Yog. The second level is Mantra Yog of sixteen limbs. The third yog is Laya yog of nine limbs and the fourth yog is Hatha Yog of six limbs. These are graduations and not cults or schools. Classical yog was maintained intact until about late 18th century. Then yog was slowly being compromised and was opened out to greater mass of people.

With the advent of 20th century, classical yog was greatly compromised and pop versions came up to appeal to a greater community and yog now remains to be a consumer product in our era.

Today, yog has only "feel-good" purpose for even those who claim to be students of yog. Another case to bow before time!

कालाय तस्मै नमः।

Prashant S. Iyengar
Pune, July 2015

Table of Contents

	Candid words from the heart	1
	Tale of the title	2
	Introduction	7
1.	Indian system of thought : Darśana	12
2.	Yoga : A Complete System on Humanics	15
3.	The source book of Yoga	20
4.	Classical Literature on Yoga	22
5.	Structure of Yoga sūtra-s	26
6.	Psychology of Yoga	36
7.	Theism of Yoga	43
8.	Cosmology of Yoga	50
9.	Teleology of Yoga	57
10.	Ontology of Yoga	59
11.	The Consummation of Yoga	62
12.	Ethico-Religious Aspects of Yoga	64
13.	Mysticism and Intuitive Mysticism of Yoga	76
14.	YOGA - A Kalpataru	98
15.	The Refutation of Yoga System in Brahmasutra	112

Candid words from the heart

Space is indeed undiscovered
by even the kings amongst fliers.

But moths and midgets, gnats and eyeflies
hesitate not to fly there.

This is a text, mystic and sacred
fit for the ramblings of sages and savants.

But here is a moth that darts upwards
in the boundless space of knowledge and wisdom.

\- *Prashant S. Iyengar*

Tale of the title

This whole compilation is woven around the *yoga sūtra-s* authored by Sage Patanjali. This work known as Patanjala *Yoga Darśana* also has a commentary by Sage Vyasa to elucidate it. The whole field of Hindu philosophy and religion is encompassed in the course of these delineations.

Hindu Philosophy and Religion has its parentage in the Vedas and have remained faithful to the parental body despite all the vicissitudes it has undergone through the ages and is still undergoing. Hindu Philosophy is the science which categorises and describes the realities of life and the realities of the Universe around us. It does this very logically, pedantically and scientifically with very little of the obscurities, so that even a scientific mind will make sense of it. It defines the Universal eternal principles and theories on the vicissitudes or phenomenalism thereof. Hindu Philosophy gives a set of minute pedantic instructions on the infinite universe to suit the spatialised human intelligence. It basically defines the trans-empirical realities which underlie the entire Universe i.e. Spirituality, Divinity and the Indestructible material entity behind all cosmic and physical phenomenalism.

Hindu Philosophy: it is a science of the macrocosm, a view of external world seen through the intuitive telescope by the great seers and a rational but devotional investigation.

Hindu religion: it means a set of instructions on a way of life which can transform the human being in its entire embodiment, into a faithful micro-replica of the macrocosm, as postulated by Hindu Philosophy.

Therefore Hindu religion is the faith which leads towards what Hindu Philosophy divulges.

It must be understood here that the Hindu view of life is not a religion that comes from a Pontiff bereft of philosophy. Hindu religion is also not a `kitchen-orthodoxy'- a mere emphasis on ritualism for ritualism's sake, nor is it an outdoor shacking and blind obedience to an external binding. Hindu Religion is the navigator which leads us along the path which Hindu philosophy divulges i.e. the path of Reality. It cares for the seeker like a mother, who looks after her child with love. It serves the seeker with everything from finite realities to the Ultimate Infinite Reality in the course of Spiritual endeavour.

Man is composed of physique and psyche. Physique means the external body and psyche comprises of the psychological forces that govern man. These forces are unique to human beings. These higher emotional, psychological and volitional aspects distinguish the human being from other creatures of the bio-world.

Hindu religion in its true sense is not just a culture of empirical mind which generates the ideal behavioural pattern of a person. It is concerned with a very high fervour, with transforming and cosmicalising every particle of human blood, every substance in the human system, and every human organism and mechanism, with cosmic energy.

The process of religious sublimation does not exclude any part or any aspect of a human being. At the same time it makes a careful, judicious discrimination in treating the various aspects of a person. The delicate aspects of a human being are handled with a light and soothing touch but the steel within the human is treated with heat and cold it requires. The means applied by religion to cosmicalise are of every kind from charming to repulsive, ravishing to obnoxious, pleasing to disgusting, gratifying to unpalatable, painful to soothing, solacious to torturing. It is true to say that steel is easier to purify than the human!

Therefore, the religious system is not merely concerned with trimming the appearance of man with refractable morality and ethicality to stand out in society, but to cosmicalise him from inside out and outside in, and from every cell to the Self.

It is by this that it tunes the physics of the human being for the cosmic symphony. By physics of the human being it means the entity composed of the five gross elements - ether, air, fire, water and earth which constitute the outer and inner organism of the human being. This tuning is essential to avoid a physical setback in the path of cosmicalisation. Religion cultures the psychics to evolve and tune the mental organism to vibrate in symphony, without mutiny. Religion deals with metapsychics to ensure that the transmigrating mind, after the end of life, does not obliterate the long process of drawing towards sublimity and cosmicalisation and that the infra mind or the eternal mind may continue imbibing the religious course. Thus, religion, with the help of its philosophy, also inducts the seeker into the knowledge of the indwelling, undislodgable, indestructible and immutable principle which is the metaphysics of the human being.

Religiosity tinges every bit of human blood, every fibre, every cell, every atom, every molecule and every corpuscular particle of the human being with the cosmic substance and natural sublimity. This brings total concordance and harmony between the human being and the cosmos with its sublime nature, which pulsates with cosmic consciousness and cosmic reality. Hindu religion, therefore, aims at bringing an excellent resonance by affecting a symphony of a sublime nature with all the human systems.

Since Hindu religion together with its philosophy is meant for the cosmicalisation of every particle of human being, the two together are considered to be the complete science of `Humanics.' Therefore this work may also serve as `A Manual on Humanics.'

This title explicitly mentions that this dissertation is a compendium of Hindu philosophy and religion. At this point it may become essential to explain the relation between Vedism and Hinduism. The obvious questions are whether the two have a relation of the nature of absolute non-difference or difference. Hinduism is not different from Vedism in so far as it is in full concordance with Vedism and owes complete fidelity to it. But Hinduism has a relation of difference with Vedism in so far as it has fallen short due to the vicissitudes it has undergone from time to time. The religion of our forefathers some tens of thousands of years ago was unquestionably different from ours of this era. Yet we belong to the same lineage as them; the faith and metaphysics are also the same.

The Vedism that has moulded itself with the essence remaining the same, has gone through innumerable adaptations, transmutations and vicissitudes. Vedism essentially generated what has now come to be called 'Hinduism'. It has assimilated all changes and has proven itself to be undislodgable by all circumstances; it remains the eternal religion. Hinduism is that faith which takes utmost pride in the primal religion, which is Vedism. It is the truest form of Vedism that exists on the surface of the earth for hundreds of centuries.

❑❑❑

Introduction

All emotions that man faces like pain and pleasure, love and hatred, devotion and profanity are on account of the mind. The mind is easily vulnerable to emotions and circumstances. It is volatile and easily provoked to fury, anxiety and excitement. Human being is more agonised by the mind than by its foes. The mental complexities grow out of proportion to such an extent that it sometimes results in split personality, and at times even landing one into an irreversible neurotic and hysterical condition. The same mind yearns for knowledge, and in its heart of hearts craves for omniscience!

A needless magnification of anguish, distress, worry, pain, sorrow, and torment victimise humanity by depriving it of placidity. Therefore, one needs to keep the mind in check for the well being of oneself and people around. Some restraint is essential to gain wisdom too. The human mind requires tender care like an infant, because it has the potential to be anything from a saint to a Satan and from wise to foolish. Although the mind is delicate, tender and complex, it can explode with catastrophic effects on the individual, society or humanity, and the bio-world at large.

The human mind has innumerable fancies and fluctuations. Man is tormented by the mercurial mind. It is the mind that makes the man excessively distressed like a naughty and a mischievous child. Man in the modern world is seen increasingly, submissively entreating his mind for peace, quietude and tranquillity. Man is seen supplicating the mind for the relinquishment of fanciful imaginings and of unduly magnified worry and anguish.

A sensitive poet is said to have expressed this feeling thus : "Alas! Being burnt up as I am with fires of the world, I take, recourse to the religion of yoga." (Y. B. 2/33).

Dissociation from pain depends upon the mind's ability to restrain its undue modulations. It also depends upon its capacity to maintain a 'low-tide' or 'no-tide' in the mind substance. This avoids catastrophic malignancies and fanciful magnifications. The mind needs to be steadfast in placidity unaffected by worldly tossing.

Yoga is development of an internal capacity to help the mind keep restrained from all fanciful, violent and turbulent radiations, and establish it in placidity. This coveted state of all-resistant and pain-proof mind is developed by rendering it into some sort of bad-conductor of psychological anguish and stress current. Such fortification could be in a way called yoga.

A commoner cherishes a pain-proof and anguish-resistant state. This is attained through an internal capacity to restrain the mind. Such internal capacities are developed by the practice of yoga principles by adherence to the yoga-cult, and by the inculcation of yoga-philosophy. It is at this point that the *yoga sūtra-s* begin declaring; 'Yoga is restraint of mental modifications.'

yogaḥ cittavṛtti nirodhaḥ I

This system of Patanjali also conjugates seemingly at the same point when the mind is irrevocably restrained in liberation, which is known as *kaivalya*. In the process, the *sūtra-s* encompass the entire human endeavour towards the summum bonum, which is religious and spiritually highest.

Now, when there is an effort to restrain all fanciful and violent flights of the mind from within oneself, the same process can be called Yoga.

Therefore, yoga becomes an indispensable path for all those who wish to get enfranchised from mental torment and beget essential, taintless, immaculate, and absolute bliss. However, yoga does not in any way mean plugging the mind or making the mind disconscious; it begins with a judicious channelisation of mental forces, and culturing of the mind-stuff. The mind needs to be known to some extent by understanding its inclinations, tendencies and propensities, before it is channelised, processed and nurtured into a desirable and virtuous disposition. It is here that the mind requires to be heated and cooled, somewhere, sometimes and in some ways. It needs to be chiselled, hammered, coaxed, soothed, enticed, persuaded, lulled, smothered, embraced and driven, but all this very judiciously, at the right time and in the right way. It is this process that cultures the mind to attain a yogic state, and the restraining capacities are engendered. The system of yoga centres around this aim, and in the process circumscribes various branches of knowledge, from the realm of the potentiality of the universe to the realm of the actuality of Universe.

The human being is made up of mind and the subject-matter of yoga has the mind in its empirical and cosmic forms. This system of thought is not merely a philosophy with excessive dialectics; it is a philosophy which makes a thorough investigation from the actuality of humanity to the potentiality of humanity and also from the potentiality of humanity to the reality of humanity. This system traverses the actuality and the potentiality of the entire living and non-living world. As far as the human mind is concerned, it bridges fictitious fancy and veritable reality en-route verisimilitude.

The cosmic mind is the seed of the cosmos and of nature, and the human mind is the seed of humanity. Man looks at cosmos or nature by being at the centre. Therefore it is necessary that the instrument of revelations, experiences and knowledge, be put in order by ridding it of ferocious and turbulent waves. Otherwise knowledge is grossly distorted. Therefore, this text begins to instruct the reader in a course of practice which removes the defects of the mind and makes it an immaculate instrument of knowledge.

The text makes a formal beginning because there are at the receiving end, seekers who yearn for release from worldly pain and pleasure dispensations. Instruction in yoga can begin for anyone who is inclined to know the science of yoga and earnestly desires wisdom. The aphorist does not stipulate as a basic qualification, qualities like placidity of mind, the capacity to curb the outgoing tendency of the senses, patience, tolerance etc. However, a seed of such qualities would be highly rewarding and would help one gallop along the path.

The true instructors of yoga, following the aphorist, are broadminded and magnanimous, assuming that the enthusiasts are ordinary but sincere aspirants on the path. Therefore, they compile the instructions from a raw beginning to the ripe end.

Yoga-sūtra-s are a systematic representation of the science of yoga. The traditions and scriptures hold that yoga has a long tradition even before Patanjali. The source of yoga, according to the scriptures, can be traced to Lord Narayana. *Mahābhārata* has recorded the instructions of Lord Narayana to his devotees- 'The luminous Hiranyagarbha, in whose praise the Vedas stand, is none other than Me. It is the same Me whom the *yogī-s* adore.' (M.Bh. 12/342/96.)

hiraṇyagarbho dyutimān ya eṣaḥ dhanyāsi stutaḥ I

yaugaiḥ sampujyate nityam sa eva hi ahaṁ bhūvi smṛtaḥ II

The *Mahābhārata* has recorded that the first principle, the Universal Principle called Hiranyagarbha, is the mentor of yoga. It tells us that 'The Hiranyagarbha' is the subject of Veda. He is the Universal Self, whom the *yogī-s* have adored (M.Bh. 12/342/96). Therefore, Patanjali *yoga-sūtra* is not the first work on yoga, but a revival, a revision, a codification and systematisation of the scattered literature on yoga. It must be deemed true that there is a long tradition of *yogācārya-s* even before Patanjali.

❑❑❑

1. Indian system of thought : *Darśana*

Darśana is understood as a system of philosophy. Philosophy is generally defined as a speculative attempt to present a systematic and complete view of reality. However, the title philosophy is very loosely conferred on any system of thought which speculates something novel, unprecedented, unusual and strange, in the realm of higher physics, metaphysics, ethics and religion, with dialectical skill. Therefore, not all philosophies of the world fulfil the requisites set out by the vague definitions of philosophy.

The Hindu *darśana-s* have been developed with more definite conventions. The edifices of *darśana* have to delineate the following aspects:

1) Epistemology (*Pramāṇa mīmāṁsā*)

This charts out the means of valid knowledge, through which the knowledge of the universe is gained.

2) Cosmology (*Viśvasaṅghaṭana mīmāṁsā*)

This spells out the universals or the unfoldment of creation and deluge, theorizing the phenomenalism.

3) Ontology (*Sattā mīmāṁsā*)

This spells out the Universals or the true entities of the Universals.

4) Teleology (*Viśva Prayojanavāda*)

This branch spells out the purpose of each principle in its ultimate analysis. It primarily stands to rule out the purposelessness of any principle or the mutation thereof in the universe.

5) Intuitive Mysticism (*Sākṣātkāra mīmāṁsā*)

This deals with the methodology for envisionment of the invisibles in the universes and the intuitive and ecstatic revelation.

6) Psychology (*Mano Vijñāna*)

This branch analyses the reaction of human mind to the universe and its knowledge. It also explains the process of gnosis (appearance of valid knowledge) the psychology of perception, illusion and the various states of consciousness.

7) Ethico-religious aspect (*dharma nīti*)

This branch spotlights the means for essential knowledge which is attained after one inculcates the moral and ethical principles. This branch provides an indispensable companion to the *mumukṣu* (the seeker of liberation) from the beginning of all human endeavors to the end of all human endeavor.

8) Theology (*Ishwara mīmāṁsā*)

Here the thought system propounds the Divinity and spells out its role in the universe. It brings out the infinite attributes and qualities of the Universal Redeemer.

The 195 brief, concise, laconic but intrinsically comprehensive statements of Patanjali encompass all these branches of knowledge. A boundless store of knowledge has been compressed in each word of each *sūtra* by the aphorist. Therefore, there is no parallel to the *yoga-sūtra-s* in the world of philosophical literature. This treatise will remain an eternal marvel particularly because this thought system that takes into account all the branches of knowledge has been articulated in only 195 statements.

❑❑❑

2. Yoga : A Complete System on Humanics

'Humanics' is the combined aspect of physics, psycho-physics, psychics, metapsychics, and meta-physics of human. The art, science and philosophy of yoga that has remedy, reformation and evolution has been bequeathed to man of any age and any era.

The curative aspect of the science of yoga has a remedy for anything from sprain in the ankle to a twist in the brain! As far as reformation is concerned, the psycho-dynamics of yoga being the most scrupulous and disciplined path has the potential of reconstituting the very nature of man. Therefore the evolution of human being is the most striking feature of the heritage of yoga. There are many instances in epics and mythology of unscrupulous men rising to heights of savant sages through yoga.

The *yama-niyama* of yoga have the capacity to reform and evolve man and to some extent also guard the man against diseases coming from over-indulgence, extravagance and intemperance. *Āsana* has come to attain the status of 'Whole Yoga' which of course, is a pitiable misconception. This is because of its capacity to set the man right from any diseases or injury coming from sprains, pulls and catches in the muscles to vital organic disorders. The health conscious people have developed a fascination for yoga mainly because of *āsana-s*. *Prāṇāyāma* too has been taken as a breathing exercise and has been conveniently deprecated for its graciousness to mend the psycho-emotional and respiratory-coronary diseases and its capacity to recuperate man's physique by mental, coronary and vascular tuning.

The higher practices of yoga are the latest natural tranquilizers for the tormented, disquiet, vexed and persecuted people of our era of speed, strain and stress. Yoga also comes to satisfy man with an intellectual quest, one with madness for rationality finds satisfaction in the science of yoga. It quenches the thirst of inquiry of an intellectual rational. This, it does by being a science with rich scholastics. Yoga as an art has over-flowing potential to more than satisfy the artiste in man. Its delicacies, finesse and points of fastidiousness are in abundance. Moreover, the art of yoga has a great grasp over the beauty in the deep unfathomable cave of heart. What is merely a void for a commoner is a rich mine of pearls and diamonds for a *yogī*, deep down in the heart. Meditation can take the *yogī* to a rapturous mood with all quietude, where the commoner draws a blank, or is dumbfounded or confounded. Yoga as a philosophy and a religious system stands indispensable for one who has an appetite for mysticism. It has a deep penetration into the mystical microcosm within. It also provides the visions in the limitless macrocosm.

As a science, yoga has made great discoveries and great strides in various branches of knowledge akin to 'Humanics' (aspects of human being). As a psychological science, yoga is just a marvel. It is the gateway for the esoterics of the science of mind of an individual to the cosmic archetypal mind of the Divinity. The human physiology has been encompassed quite thoroughly in the science of yoga where *bandha-s* and *kriyā-s* have some symbolism as exoterics to define the esoterics of physiology. The esoterics of physiology are described in some *Hatha-yogic* and *Tantric* texts. The concept of *cakra-s* (plexus) conveys that the chakras are vital physio-psycho-neuro junctions in the cerebro-spinal system and with the interactions of vital air, they release unusual energies and change the mental state conducive to yoga practices. Many *yogīc* practices reform the human system by activating or hibernating those physio-psycho-neuro junctions.

Modern medicine has corroborated facts of esoteric physiology spelled out in yoga texts of great antiquity. What the *yogī-s* knew in the remote past, science has revealed at the turn of the twentieth century. The mental conditioning and culturing that yoga speaks of, is through the profound and scientific knowledge that it has of some vital conditioners of glands and plexi, or the psycho-neuro centres of physiology. The investigation that has been made by ancient *yogī-s* of the cerebrospinal tract, the most vital anatomical, physiological, psychological and neurological part of man is just incredible and marvellous. Patanjali's articulation of the knowledge of the human body by profound meditation on the navel, spells out the science of embryology known to *yogī-s*. He relates thirst and hunger to the physio-psycho-neuro junction at the throat, which reveals the knowledge of esoteric physiology of our ancient yogis.

The concept of *pañca-kośa* (developed in *Vedānta* and yoga) speak of *annamaya, prāṇamaya, manomaya, vijñānamaya* and *ānandamaya* sheaths of the body which are the esoterics of physiology not yet fully understood by the modern sciences of anatomy, physiology and neurology. The ancient *Garbha Upaniṣad* is the proof of an advanced state of knowledge of anatomy and physiology without the mechanical insights provided by X-rays and endoscopies of today. The *Upaniṣad-s* also have so often spoken of countless *nāḍi-s* and their roles. The *Tantra* and *Hatha-yoga* texts have posited that all physiology has its switch house in the brain which concurs with the view of modern medicine.

The yoga postures, based on various species in the bio-world, entitle yoga to be called a bio-engineering subject. The *iḍā-piṅgaḷā-suṣumnā* concept developed in *Hathayoga* texts may be called the bio-electricals of physiology as they deal with positive, negative and neutral currents.

The *yoga-sūtra-s* have gone into the physics of the cosmos in postulating the theory of evolution of *prakṛti*. They have dealt with cosmology which is an important branch of any Indian Philosophical system. They have also made a mention of their own scientific processes to investigate astronomy which is infinite around us. The *sūtra-s* say that by profound meditation (*saṁyama*) on the sun, the knowledge of the astral planes ensues. By profound meditation on the moon, the knowledge of the starry system ensues. And by the same on the pole-star, comes knowledge of the velocities and movements of stars and planets. The *yogī*'s free entry into any field or branch of knowledge is spelled out in the *yoga-sūtra-s* (3/32.)

The *yoga-sūtra-s* as a system of religion and philosophy has delineated epistemology, cosmology, ontology, teleology, theology and science of religion.

Patanjali in the first chapter says that, with practice of ethico-religious principles of yoga comes absence or removal of disease, languor, doubt, heedlessness, sloth, passion, illusion or deceptive convictions, delusion of goals, fall from attainments, pain, despair, infirmness in the body and spasmodism of breath, etc. This ensures physical, physiological, intellectual, and spiritual wealth to the practitioner of yoga, which is verily the summum bonum of all spiritual endeavours. Nothing remains to be attained by a man when he is graced with all these gifts. This particular *yoga-sūtra* in a way defines a perfect man, a complete being and a human par-excellence.

It will be appropriate to mention that the Bhagwad *Gītā* too holds the view that yoga is a complete science and a Brahma *vidyā*. Each chapter ends with a colophon as follows :

Thus ends __________ (chapter named) ____________ in the dialogue between Sri Krishna and Arjuna on the yoga included in the science of Brahmin in the Upanishad sung by the Lord.

❑❑❑

3. The source book of Yoga

Yoga literature has remained widely scattered in ancient Hindu book i.e. *Veda, Upaniṣad*, *Smṛti*, *Itihāsa* and *Purāṇa-s* etc.

The yoga tradition holds that the first and the foremost text on yoga is the *Hiraṇyagarbha* yoga. This text has been lost to us. It is however believed that Patanjali *yoga-sūtra* is based on this text. However, a doubt is raised to the veracity of the same. Since the text is totally unavailable to us, it requires to be proved that the *yoga-sūtra* is faithful to the first text on yoga.

Pañcarātra is the text revered by the Vaiṣṇavites. It has been extolled in the *Mahābhārata* as a five-day discourse by Lord Narayana to his distinguished devotees in His abode, Vaikuntha. The *Pañcarātara* is composed of many books called as *saṁhitā-s*. One of these *saṁhitā-s* is the famous *Ahirbudhnya saṁhitā*. This text has provided some edifices and relics of *Hiraṇyagarbha* yoga. This helps one to draw a parallel between *yoga-sūtra* and the first and foremost text on yoga called *Hiraṇyagarbha* yoga. It is evident from the *saṁhitā* that the first text on yoga also mentioned yoga of eight limbs which are referred to by the *sūtra-s* (Ah. Bu. Sa. 3/607). It has also classified the eight limbs of yoga as external and internal as demarcated by Patanjali (Ah. Bu. 13/28). Therefore it is irrefutable that Patanjali *yoga sūtra-s* are completely faithful to the earliest text on yoga and that the *sūtra-s* are merely representation and schematisation of the Hiranyagarbha-yoga, and all the scattered references to yoga in the scriptures.

Patanjali has done a commendable service by codifying the science of yoga and putting it in a frame-work that every classical Hindu philosophy demands. He has schematised the subject-matter of yoga and has codified it with the fewest, but immaculate words. The whole boundless store of knowledge has been encapsulated in just 195 aphorisms. (which are not even 195 sentences)

❑❑❑

4. Classical Literature on Yoga

Upaniṣad-s went all in for the praise of yoga and reinstated the glory of yoga that was lost. *Mahābhārata* has more than sufficient material on yoga. No *purāṇa* has overlooked yoga. It is no exaggeration but a reality that each *purāṇa* has a chapter or two on yoga. A special mention of Vishnu *purāṇa* here is very tempting. The last chapter of this *purāṇa* overflows with a discourse on yoga in a dialogue form.

Amongst the practical *Upaniṣad-s, Katha* has defined yoga. The *Śvetāśvatāra* has described meditation. There is a set of *Upaniṣad-s*, called Yoga *Upaniṣad-s* which have been completely devoted to yoga. These are :

1) Yoga *Chuḍāmaṇi Upaniṣad*
2) *Mahā Upaniṣad*
3) Yoga *Kuṇḍalinī Upaniṣad*
4) *Dhyāna Sindhu Upaniṣad*
5) *Saubhāgya Lakṣmi Upaniṣad*
6) *Amṛtānanda Upaniṣad*
7) *Nādabindu Upaniṣad*
8) *Śāṇḍilya Upaniṣad*
9) *Darśana Upaniṣad*

10) *Maṇḍala Brahmaṇa Upaniṣad*

There is also a famous text on yoga ascribed to *yogī* Yajnavalkya, the composer of Sathapatha Brahmana and chief speaker instructor of the famous *Brihadaranyaka Upaniṣad*. This text of Yajnavalkya is remembered as *Yogī Yajnavalkya Smriti*. This is an indispensable text for the students of yoga. Instructions on yoga are also abundantly found in the *śānti parva* of *Mahābhārata* as well as in the *purāṇa-s*. This set of yoga-literature is pre-Patanjali literature.

The yoga-literature is therefore to be divided into two parts :

1) Pre Patanjali

2) Post Patanjali

The *yoga-sūtra* forms an important land-mark in the yoga-literature. It was for the first time that the subject matter of yoga was philosophised systematically with no hyperboles, exaggerations and rhetoric. The seers of *Upaniṣads*, *purāṇa-s*, and *Mahābhārata* have gone into raptures because no praise was sufficient for this marvelous mystic science.

Although the yoga literature is widely scattered in ancient Hindu texts and Universal Literature - the Vedas, it was first arranged in a systematic form by Sage Patanjali. The construction of *yoga-sūtra-s*, though contracted and squeezed into a mere 195 statements, each word in the *sūtra* is impregnated with greater implicit than explicit value. Each *sūtra* throbs with significance, instructions, and suggestions with high value.

It is because of Patanjali, that yoga has a berth in the Hindu *Darśana* with the bare minimum aphorisms. The following table gives the idea of compactness of *yoga-sūtra* compared to the other orthodox philosophers and their philosophies :

TEXT	AUTHOR	NUMBER OF SUTRAS
Yoga sūtra-s	Patanjali	195
Nyāya sūtra-s	Gautama	530
Vaiṣeśika sūtra-s	Kanade	371
Brahma sūtra-s	Badrayana	535
Mimāṁsā sūtra-s	Jaimini	2644
Saṁkhya sūtra-s	Kapila	524

The post-*yoga-sūtra* literature is led by the revered Vyasa. He composed the *Yoga-bhāṣya*, a commentary on *yoga-sūtra*. The yoga tradition strongly believes that this Vyasa is none other than Veda-Vyasa or Dvaipayana-Vyasa, the prolific writer of Vedic literature. This Vyasa, the son of Parasara and great grandson of Vasistha, rearranged the Vedas in the manner in which they have come down to us. The eighteen *purāṇa-s* are ascribed to his name. The *Mahābhārata*, the mine of knowledge is also authored by him.

Vyasa's commentary was subjected to interpretations and elucidations from time to time. There are elucidations of *Yoga-Bhāṣya* such as:

1) Vachaspati Mishra's Gloss (Tattva Vaisaradi)
2) Sankārācārya's *bhāṣya* Vivarana
3) *Vijñāna* Bhikṣhu's Vartika
4) *Vṛtti* of Bhāva Ganesha
5) *Vṛtti* of Nagoji Bhatta and so on.

Following is the list of standard classical literature on *Yoga Darśana* ;

1) *Yoga-sūtra-s* of Patanjali (pre-historic times)

2) *Yoga-bhāṣya* of Vyāsa (pre-historic times)

3) *Yoga-bhāṣya*-Vivarnam of Shankaracharya (8th century)

4) Tattva Vaisharadi of Mishra (10th century)

5) Bhoja *vṛtti* of Rajamartanda Bhoja (10th century)

6) *Yoga* Vartika of *Vijñānaa* Bhikshu (16th century)

7) *Yoga*-Dipika of Bhave Ganesha (17th century)

8) Chāyā *vṛtti* of Nagoji Bhatt (17th century)

9) Maniprabhā of Narayanayati (17th century)

10) *Yoga* Sudhākara of Sadashivendra (18th century)

❑❑❑

5. Structure of *Yoga sūtra-s*

The *yoga-sūtra-s* have been arranged in four quarters of four chapters. These are named as:

a) *Samādhi pāda* - Chapter on Trance (51)

b) *Sādhana pāda* - Chapter on Practice (55)

c) *Vibhūti pāda* - Chapter on Attainments (54)

d) *Kaivalya pāda* - Chapter on Liberation (34)

The *Samādhi pāda* makes a formal beginning by defining yoga. Yoga being restraint of mental modifications, the aphorist mentions five mental modifications which are either afflictive (drawing the seeker away from wisdom) or non-afflictive (drawing the seeker towards wisdom). The five mental modifications called *citta vṛtti* arc valid cognition, illusion, verbal delusion, dreamless sleep and memory. The valid cognition can be three fold i.e. direct perception, inference and testimonial cognition. These *citta vṛtti-s* are defined and characterised.

Yoga being a trance, by affecting inhibition for externalisation in the consciousness and thereby in the outer senses, the science of yoga theorised that all five *citta vṛtti-s* are to be restrained for such a state. The means for such a restraint are *abhyāsa* (practice) and *vairāgya* (thirstlessness). *Abhyāsa* is a relentless and ardent but reverential attempt to abate the super mercurial mental forces. Any effort from within to check the mind from ramblings is technically called as *abhyāsa*. *Vairāgya* is said to be thirstlessness for all terrestrial and extra-terrestrial objects.

Commensurate with the application, adoption, inculcation of the means, which are *abhyāsa-vairāgya, samādhi* or trance actualises in the *citta*. The mental forces are made to retrace the consciousness. This expands the characteristics of the trance in the consciousness called as *samādhi dharma*. In accordance with the appearance of characteristic of trance in the consciousness, the trance of various modes actualises progressively. The aphorist at this point mentions four phases of *samādhi* viz.

a) *VITARKA ANUGATA* - *citta* obsessed with gross metaphysical-metapsychical matter.

b) *VICĀRA ANUGATA* - *citta* obsessed with subtle metaphysical matter.

c) *ĀNANDA ANUGATA* - obsessed by ecstasy of bliss coming on account of retrocession

d) *ASMITĀ ANUGATA* - unified in a subjectivistic state whereby the consciousness is compressed in the principle of 'I'.

These four *samādhi-s* are called as *saṁprajñāta samādhi* because they are cognitive trance on account of occurring of some revelations. All the mystic, intuitive and ecstatic revelations for the *yogī* come forth in the cognitive trance called *saṁprajnāta samādhi.*

The aphorist mentions that the *vairāgya* is of two levels, the lower and the higher. The lower level of *vairāgya* brings about the cognitive trance, while the highest *vairāgya* grants the ultra-cognitive trance called *asaṁprajnāta samādhi*. It is in this trance that there is a total and grand restraint of mental modifications. In other words, during this trance the seer or the *Puruṣa* or the Self, is free from mental hurricane.

The ultra-cognitive trance is attained if the practice is according to the set of practices, shown in the ethico-religious aspects of *yoga-sūtra-s*. They are to be practised with faith (*śraddhā*), vigour (*vīrya*), memory imprints (*smṛti*), trancive practices (*samādhi*) and discernment (*prajñā*). The intensities in the practices and thirstlessness determine the gestation period in yoga. However, the dedication and devotion to the Lord (*Ishwara*) accelerates the process. Thus, propounding of an entity called *Ishwara*, necessitates the aphorist to mention the infinite qualities and powers of *Ishwara*, which he does with bare minimum words. The dedication and devotion to the Lord plays an invaluable role in the pursuit of *yoga Sādhana* from a raw beginning to the ripe end. It is basically because, God is omnipotent and highly magnanimous to enfranchise the seeker from all sorts of impediments, blockades and obstacles. These obstacles as summarised by the aphorist are :

a) Disease *(vyādhi)*

b) Languor *(styāna)*

c) Doubt *(saṁśaya)*

d) Heedlessness *(pramāda)*

e) Sloth *(ālasya)*

f) Sensuality *(avirati)*

g) Mistaken notion *(bhrāntidarśana)*

h) Non-attainment of state for consolidation *(alabdhabhūmikatva)*

i) regression or instability *(anavasthitatva)*

These impediments are accompanied by pains (*duḥkha*), despair (*daurmanasya*), infirmity (*aṅgamejayatva*) in limbs of the body and loss of rhythm in the breathing *(śvāsapraśvāsa)*.

Even with this set of impediments being quite a formidable array of opponents, the seeker is instructed not to loose heart, but to continue the practices and pursuits with unabated zeal and zest. There should be no deviation or distraction, but as the aphorist says, *tatpratiṣedhārtham ekatattva abhyāsaḥ* meaning unaltered, unalternated and undeviated practice.

In order to combat the quite formidable combination of antagonists, the aphorist expects the seeker to cultivate and develop some principles and beget a steadfast character and placidity of mind. This forms the mind culturing practices of yoga called *cittaparikarma* (cleansing of the mind).

The means are such as

a) cultivating friendliness, compassion, complacency and indifference towards happiness, misery, virtue and vice respectively of other people.

b) a particular breathing pattern.

c) a higher sense activity peculiar to yoga.

d) a mental figuration of luminous but a sorrowless state.

e) a mental figuration of thirstlessness.

f) mental culturing by recalling dreams where one has experienced transfigurations of one's attitudes, or understanding and inducing the gradual mental retirement coming in sleep.

g) meditation on deity of one's liking.

By above practices one attains a capacity to make any subject from the subtlest ultra-matter to grossest matter as object for meditation and reveal the same. These revelations occur on account of what yoga psychology calls *samāpatti*. This is the state where the *citta* attains an identity with the object of meditation. When proficiency is attained in *samāpatti* the seeker is fit to experience subjective luminosity (*adhyātmaprasādaḥ*) and from this ensues a faculty of essential cognition (*ṛtaṁbharā prajñā*). The perception, revelation, and conviction developed by this faculty are incomparable, on account of their flawlessness.

This exalted knowledge helps the *yogī* reap superior impressions (*prajñā saṁskāra*) whereby the *yogī* gallops to the goal i.e. the liberation-the Brahmanisation.

The second chapter unveils to the neophyte, the basics and preliminaries of yoga practices. The authentic practices of yoga are characterised as *Kriyā-yoga*. *Kriyā-yoga* is a composite practice of '*tapas*' (austerities), *svādhyāya* (self-study and study of spiritual sciences and texts) and '*Iśvarapraṇidhāna*' (the natural disposition to begin, carry out and end any work for God and offer the same with its fruits to God). This requires enrichment of the theistic and religious consciousness.

Inculcating the principles of *Kriyā-yoga* smoothens the path to *samādhi* and also attenuates the afflictions, called as *kleśa-s*. The afflictions are meta-psychical illusions, which roll the human being from birth to death and death to birth, as well as rotate the human beings in countless species of living and non-living creation. These afflictions are five:

1) *Avidyā*: perverse knowledge

2) *Asmitā*: egoism

3) *Rāga*: attachment

4) *Dveśa*: aversion

5) *Abhiniveśa*: self benediction or clinging to life

These *kleśa-s*, if subtle and attenuated, would be totally destroyed, when the *yogī* is liberated from the contact of *prakṛti*. The grosser and workable *kleśa-s*, however, may be suppressed by meditative practices before they are attenuated.

The meta-psychical illusions are causal for transmigration birth and experience during the lifetime. The beings are rotated by time in the fuel of afflictions which are self-generating.

Be it pain or pleasure, the wise man comes to resolve that all the painful, pleasurable and delusive experiences are ultimately painful in so far as they provide motivation to roast and rotate the beings in the experiences of the mundane world and wean away one from the summum bonum of the spiritual endeavour. The wise is truly agonised by the experiences of the mundane world. The agony is further aggravated by the fact that the three *guṇa-s* work contrarily. This enmeshes the beings and ties them firmly in the mundane world.

As all the empirical, psychological and physical experiences of the nature of pain, pleasure and delusion, are ultimately painful, and because the pain must be abandoned, a theorem is articulated that, the pain which is in store is fit to be avoided. The aphorist then proceeds to investigate the cause of pain, the nature of freedom and means of freedom from such pain. It is at this point that, the aphorist presents a scheme for freedom from pain. This verily is the renowned *Aṣṭāṅga yoga,* the yoga of eight limbs.

These eight limbs are :

1) *yama* : (Restraints) :

a) *ahiṁsā* - non-injury

b) *satya* - veracity

c) *asteya* - non stealing

d) *brahmacarya* - celibacy, continence

e) *aparigraha* - non-hoarding

2) *niyama* : (Observances) :

a) *śauca* - cleanliness

b) *santoṣa*- contentment

c) *tapa* - austerity

d) *svādhyāya* - studiousness

e) *Ishwara praṇidhāna* - feeling and inclination to incorporate theos (theism) in actions.

3) *āsana* : Posture

4) *prāṇāyāma* : Control over life-force

5) *pratyāhāra* : Abstraction, withdrawing the senses from their objects.

6) *dhāraṇā* : Concentration

7) *dhyāna* : Meditation

8) *samādhi* : Trance

It is also in this chapter that the aphorist delineates on the metaphysical aspect of yoga system. The system holds that ontologically there are two entities in the Universe viz.

1) *puruṣa*: (conscious principle)

2) *prakṛti*: (unconscious principle)

prakṛti is postulated to be the primordial substance of the intrinsic nature of the *guṇa-s*. These *guṇa-s* correspond as listed below:

	Sattva	**Rajas**	**Tamas**
Physical	Luminosity	Activity	Intertia
Mental	Placidity or pleasure	Turbulence or pain	Delusion
Psychological	Intelligence	Craze	Delirium

As against *prakṛti, puruṣa* is exclusively a principle of consciousness (*cinmātra*) completely distinct from the *guṇa-s* of *prakṛti.* The *Ishwara* of Patanjali is a distinct, special *puruṣa* who is (*ekamevādvitiya*) the one without second.

It is here that the second chapter articulates the cosmology, propounded by the *Sāṁkhya-yoga* system. The aphorist states that, the whole cosmological unfoldment is from the primordial matter. This unfoldment is effected in four phases:

1) Unmarked phase (potentiality)

2) Marked phase (seed stage)

3) Unparticularised phase (infra-atomic stage of the mind and matter)

4) Particularised phase (actualised creation of mind and matter)

In short, the second chapter is packed with metaphysics, cosmology, teleology and ethico-religious principles of yoga system.

The third chapter deals with the definition of concentration, meditation and trance. The trance which is of cognitive nature is the womb of all excellence of a *yogī.* This trance engenders the expanse of knowing power, sense power and bio-power of yoga. The aphorist presents the psychological process of the trance by mentioning three fold modifications of the consciousness for the trance. Incidentally aphorist also states that the whole phenomenal creation also undergoes similar three-fold modifications. This spells out the process of cosmological unfoldment of Universe. This chapter makes a fascinating delineation on expanse in the powers of *yogī* who attains the stage of *samādhi*.

The powers subjected to expanse are:

1) *jñāna śakti* (power of knowing)

2) *citta śakti* (power of consciousness)

3) *prāṇa śakti* (power of bio-force)

4) *śarīra śakti* (power of physique)

5) *indriya śakti* (power of inner, outer senses)

The chapter culminates by mentioning that the exalted wisdom ensuing from the *samādhi* takes the *yogī* to the peak of spiritual endeavour i.e. the Final Release.

Fourth chapter accounts for certain meta-psychical processes. It provides very rational answers to questions such as the cause of transmigrations, the trans-empirical laws of regulating the fruitions of actions, and determination and effectualisation and rebirth in its class, style and span. The chapter also defines subliminal tendencies (*vāsanā*) which is locus of all behaviours and actions.

The chapter also gives a finishing touch to the metaphysics, by providing some finer points in the process of Creation. The chapter also has successfully disproved the basic counter arguments of heterodox schools, which reject the very entity of the permanent principle, immutable principle, the Self. It also disproves the stand of idealists that whole creation is false, illusory and nugatory. Without answering the nihilist, momentarist, agnostic, idealist and pan-illusionist, who try to hit the orthodox philosophy at the very source, the position of the metaphysics, cosmology, teleology and ontology, held by Patanjali would have been blasted to total annihilation by a dialectical dynamite. Therefore this chapter is of great importance to fortify all the basic tenets of the Philosophy of Patanjali.

The chapter culminates with articulation and description of the process in which the *yogī* makes a grand departure from this phenomenal world comprising of terrestrial and extra-terrestrial planes. The *yogī* is said to be casting out the psychic and astral bodies for the grand disembodiment and attain Brahmanisation.

❑❑❑

6. Psychology of Yoga

Exclusion of mind from the subject-matter of yoga is like talking about the ocean without the mention of water. At the outset, one would know that what is conceived by psychology in Indian system of thought is poles apart from what is conceived by western psychology. Western psychology is generally understood as a study of behaviourism, which it basically is. It has tended to be parochial, for it is obsessed with the instincts of bio-world in general and humanity in particular. The whole of western psychology has for some reason been obsessed by the sullied sub-conscious basic tendencies of the human being.

Although Indian psychology also deals with reactions of the mind to experience, sensations and knowledge, it is altogether on a different footing. Basically this is because it holds that even the empirical mind is spatialisation and delimitation of the cosmic mind. The cosmic mind being a subject-matter of metaphysics, psychology becomes not only dependent on metaphysics but also an integral part of Hindu metaphysics. Therefore, Indian psychology did not evolve as an independent science. This does not mean that the subject of psychology was deprecated by Indian thinkers. The fact is that the subject-matter of psychology is the empirical mind. But it is not altogether a different substance from the cosmic mind. And further, the empirical mind has its origin in the cosmic mind. Since the cosmic principles are investigated by metaphysics, psychology was treated as a para-metaphysical aspect and hence not treated independently. It may be noted that an independent treatment to psychology would be a mal-investigation. Western psychology never takes into account the root mind which is cosmic mind, the subject-matter of metaphysics, but gets stuck in the subconscious mind of the psyche.

Psychology being an integral part of all *Darśana-s*, has had multitudinous treatment from each system. However, the psychology evolved in *Yoga-Darśana* has stood out with marked distinction. Indian psychology never had a raw deal like its western counterpart; firstly, because Indians traced the root of human mind in the cosmic mind, unlike the westerners, who traced it into the sullied subconscious plane. Moreover, Indian psychology has a welcome touch of religious principles, theology and a berth in metaphysics of *darśana-s*. The west evolved a psychology that was castigated from such rich companies and was distorted by the sullied subconscious garbage.

Indian psychology has also analysed the reaction of the human mind to the universe and its knowledge. It has spelled out the process of gnosis (psychology of perception). It has also analysed the psychology of illusion and hallucination. The yoga psychology has gone beyond what has been mentioned in the foregoing. It has analysed the mental processes and has evolved schemes of culturing of the mind by understanding the various states of consciousness. The state of consciousness is the shape of mind-stuff as an activity potential behind psycho-mental-senso-motor activity. It is also a receptacle of impressions of all psycho-senso-motor activity. Basically any state of consciousness has a stark nature of vibrating sentient force, and it forms proto-structure of every individual. Therefore, it may be called as hypostatisation of an individual at the psychic level.

The man reacts to the experiences with following set of states of consciousness.

1) Exhibitive consciousness: It is the one that inclines and engages the person excessively into the business of life with flamboyance. This also magnifies ego, hypocrisy, pride and showmanship.

2) Inhibitive consciousness: This makes one retrace from the worldly life and excessive business life. This is developed wrongly out of despair, dejection and frustration, but is rightly developed when accompanied by intellection and thirstlessness.

3) Enduring consciousness: This subjects the person to undergo the experience of pain and pleasure and also helps to gain empirical knowledge.

4) Retributive consciousness: This is developed out of abashment and remorse for the sins committed. Thereafter the expiatory acts are also undertaken willingly to wash off sins and effect self-regulation.

5) Reactionary consciousness: This brings forth the attachment to and lust for the pleasurable, and hate and aversion for the painful. This roils the person, down into the vicious valley of sin.

The above five states spell out human reaction to sensation, knowledge and experience. Following is the set of consciousness which is evolved in the course of *yogīc* pursuit:

1) Physical consciousness - This should not be mistaken for body consciousness, which is an outcome of Narcissus-complex and which is a very epicurean state. But this is an awareness that shoots from every cell in the body by being intelligised and animated with life force. This helps the yoga-practitioner to get a subjective sensitivity in various parts of the body.

2) Physiological consciousness - This helps the yoga practitioner to attain keen sensitivity in the inner organism comprising of vital streams and physio-psycho-neuro centres.

3) Mental consciousness - It is a sort of perceptive vision of one's own mind, very much required for self-analysis and self study in the heuristic aspects of yoga.

4) Intellectual consciousness or cerebral-cortical consciousness - This again is peculiar to yoga-psychology, where, by increase and decrease in the density of cerebral-cortical psychological flux, the *yogī* effects hypo-active or hyper-active states in the various physiological parts of body with the interaction of the vital force (prāṇa).

5) Psychological consciousness - It is a state peculiar to mental practices of yoga. Here, the practitioner makes one's own senses and brain as objects in various acts of yoga, and ascertains their physiological and psychological states and then learns to make necessary modifications in them through physio-psycho-neuro bio-interactions.

6) Ego consciousness - This is the envisionment of the cosmic substance in one's own heart. It is the locus of all

internal and external voluntary activities. This vision comes by a centripetal movement of the mind-stuff.

7) Spiritual consciousness - It is an inclination to go after in search of the principle of consciousness which is eternal, immutable, immovable, formless, spiritual principle.

8) Theistic consciousness - Though this is an intellectual conviction of existence of Divinity or a mental belief in God, nevertheless a springboard for virtues and spiritual evolution. It is a thickly insulated deism. Therefore deistic impulses are not capable of being surfaced. It distinguishes an atheist from a temporal materialist profane.

9) Religious consciousness - Here the spiritual consciousness gets dis-insulated from deism and becomes capable of firing electrical impulses from neurons to muscles, bones and skin endings of a person. The emotional impulses are developed on the theistic consciousness at intellectual level. It is an ecstatic impulse chemically and electrical impulse neurologically, psychologically and physically. It is the God-intoxicated state of mystic saints.

10) Unity consciousness - The vision that the spiritual principle in all the beings is one and identical and that in ultimate analysis, there is no ground to differentiate and discriminate amongst them.

11) Trance consciousness - The crystal like taintless consciousness in *samādhi*.

These states are subjectivistic, coming in retrocession. The yoga-psychology is not as much concerned with normalization of subnormal tendencies as it is with transcendence and transfiguration of normal tendencies.

Yoga aims at wisdom, through knowledge process as well as intuitive mysticism and trancive revelations. Therefore, it characterises another set of consciousness such as:

1) Intuitive consciousness - The development of intuitive faculty which opens out entry for the *yogī* in any field of knowledge and grants instantaneous knowledge by flash of consciousness.

2) Ecstatic consciousness - It is the ecstatic bliss that comes in introcession for a *yogī*.

3) Revelatory consciousness - It is the development of faculty of essential knowledge called *ṛtaṁbharā prajna* (described in Y.S. 1/48). Through it, the *yogī* gets the envisionment of all that is subtle, veiled and remote.

Yoga system is primarily practical in approach. Therefore, all the means of practices are psychologically analysed.

Psychology of *samādhi* is the basic field of investigation in the yoga system. It rationally presents a physico-psycho scheme towards that end. It mentions a mental scheme for attaining capacity for trance (*samādhi*) in the Sutras -1/33 to 1/39. The psychology of trance is explained in *samāpatti* (1/41 to 1/46). In the third chapter there is psychology of mental restraint, called three-fold *citta-pariṇāma* (3/9 to 3/12).

The second chapter opens out with *Kriyā-yoga* to mention metapsychology of yoga. The afflictions (*kleśa-s*) find source not in the empirical mind but the greater mind. Those are ceaselessly influencing all beings from time without beginning. The *avidyā* which is perverse knowledge, is not psycho-temporal or temporal-intellectual perversion, but is meta-psychic illusion. The same chapter while dealing with *karma vipāka* (fruition of action) shows the relation between psychology and meta-psychology. It may be understood here that psychology only deals with the movement of mind in the living being, while metapsychology also speaks of transmigrating mind which is eternal.

The fourth chapter while dealing with transmigration of subtle body speaks of meta-psychical evolution for change in class at the time of rebirth. It may be pointed out here that the meta-psychic substance is the same in all the creatures from infernal worlds to celestial worlds.

The third chapter deals with the branch of parapsychology by describing the *yogīc* powers like Extra Sensory Perception and so on.

The fourth chapter establishes that the mind too is material because it is nothing other than the three *guṇa-s*.

❑❑❑

7. Theism of Yoga

The *yoga darśana* stands distinctly separate from *Sāṁkhya*-philosophy typified in the *Sāṁkhya-kārika* of Īśvarakrisna. It is on this account that the yoga system came to be called *Seśvara Sāṁkhya*, meaning theistic *Sāṁkhya*.

The theism of yoga is not in anyway to propound a religious idealism represented by polytheism, monotheism or pantheism etc. Nor, is it a compromise with deistic people, or a move to gain popularity among the general public particularly, because the *Vaidika-s* were deistic and religious people.

The *Ishwara* of Patanjalas is an ontological or a metaphysical principle; the one without second. This *Ishwara* as explicitly described in the *sūtra* is *puruṣa viśeṣa* (special being) untouched by the vehicles of afflictions, actions and fruitions (Y.S. 1/24). His supremacy is par excellence, hence the unexceedable power and glory. In stating the supremacy of *Ishwara*, Veda is mutually testified. (Y.B. 1/24). The commentator makes the position of Patanjalas clear that they too hold *Ishwara* as the source of the Vedas. This is the relation between Veda and God as held by *Vaidika-s*. *Ishwara*, according to the aphorist is not merely omniscient but, in Him the seed of omniscience is unexceedable (Y.S. 1/25). The compassion of

Ishwara knows no bounds, according to Vyasa. Vyasa towards the end of comment on 1/25 tells us that the consummating knowledge is dispensed by God. *Ishwara* is the first and foremost of all preceptors besides being the eternal preceptor not being limited by time (Y.S. 1/26). *Ishwara*, according to Patanjalas is the Highest Entity by being denotative of *prāṇava* (*āuṁ*) (Y.S. 1/27). At this point, it is intended to make clear that the postulation of *Ishwara* by Patanjalas is not a philosophical expediency, nor is it a secondary postulate. The status accorded to *Ishwara* in the yoga philosophy is also not titular or formal.

Ishwara is attained by the devotee through the *prāṇava-japa* with the intrinsic purport of the *prāṇava* manifest in the heart of the devotee (Y.S. 1/28). This *japa* is not merely repetition of '*āuṁ*' orally or mentally but a mystic practice of yoga-religion, making the '*āuṁ*' as the means as well as the end. Yoga, as VYASA says, ensues from *prāṇava* and *prāṇava* ensues from yoga (Y.B. 1/28).

The section of *yoga sūtra* dealing with *Ishwara* has been subjected to severe criticism more often than not, in the dialectics of Indian philosophical systems. This is because of the manner in which this section appears to be is a little superficial. It appears to be suggesting that the devotion to *Ishwara* quickens the attainment of ultra-cognitive trance called *asaṁprajñāta samadhi*. This section commences thus:

The ultra-cognitive trance is proximate for those whose consciousness of supremacy is keen and intense. This intense supremacy of consciousness reaps the said trance in the quickest possible and shortest time (Y.S. 1/21, 22). Alternately, the *sūtra* suggests the devotion for *Ishwara* may also reap the end-yoga in quickest and shortest time (Y.S. 1/23). Critics argue here that *Ishwara* in the *yoga-sūtra-s* comes as an alternate means for success, which, as a matter of fact, does not honour God but deprecates Him!

The above judgement is immature and far from being a reality. It is a failure in understanding the conclusion of the section on *Ishwara*, in its explicit and implicit sense. The aphorist undoubtedly holds Him as the Universal redeemer, when he mentions that the Lord dismisses and dislodges the obstacles that block the path of seeker towards the goal (Y.S. 1/30). If at all a question at this point is raised, it will be only by the connoisseur critic, that the *Ishwara* for Patanjalas is not the Goal but He is merely a path-clearer. This is because *Ishwara* has been stated to be clearing obstacles from the path of seeker towards the Goal. Let us analyse and sort out the problem posed by the prima-facie view.

The prima-facie argument is thus:-

In the mention that *prāṇava japa* obliterates all the obstacles in the path of a yogi; the major goal of yogi clearly seems to be ultra-cognitive trance and *kaivalya*. The obstacles in the path are disease, languor, doubt, sloth, heedlessness in *sādhanā*, sensuality, delusive notions, lack of progress, regress, sorrow, dejection, infirmity in body for yogic practices and lack of control on vital forces (breath). The yoga practitioner wants a super path-clearer or super pilot to obliterate the formidable foes and make the path void of thorns and roughs. It is then that the yoga practitioner prostrates at the feet of the Lord.

Let us go on to encounter the above accusation of the opponent that God has been relegated with the job of serving the *yogī* to clear his path. And that, the induction of an *Ishwara* in the yoga-system is a convenience-measure and a formality. Their first conviction is that the goal of *yogī* is *kaivalya* and they take it as something different than the ultimate goal spelled out in *Upaniṣad,* which is Braḥmaṇisation. They seem to hold *kaivalya* as an acosmic state ---- What is this *kaivalya then*?

Is it anything different than the summum bonum of all spiritual endeavour explained in the Upanishads?

Let the opponent spell out the difference in two statements:

1) I want to die, and

2) I don't want to live.

Similar are the two statements :

1) I want liberation / release / *kaivalya* and

2) I want God attainment/Highest beatitude / Braḥmaṇisation

kaivalya means a complete cessation of sorrow (not in the temporal or psychological sense but in philosophical sense). The absolute release from sorrow is nothing but culmination of highest beatitude. Since the highest beatitude lies in God attainment, the complete enfranchisement from all sorts of sorrows is implied. Therefore it is a sheer jugglery in arguing that the two things viz.

1) complete enfranchisement from sorrow and

2) attainment of God

are two different and distinct goals.

Therefore the accusation of prima-facie view that the Patanjalas cherish something other than God-attainment is a baseless and unfounded accusation.

Secondly, the prima-facie view considers that there is a highest honour to God in holding Him as exclusively of a category of an ultimate Goal. They sense a deprecation of God in rendering Him as the instrument for goal as well. They seem to hold God as the Lord of the seventh Heaven whose place is unsurmountable, and that, to reach that Royalty one needs the assistance of an apostle or a middleman or a divine messenger. The Lord is not a Royalty in the heavens, only concerned with commanding respect for His physical glory and charisma. They need to be told that, God despite all His incalculable and insurmountable glories is ever the seeker after earnest and fond devotion from His Creation. His craving, yearning and eagerness for the call of His devotees are ever intense. His ears are ever keen erect and alert; ever awaiting to receive the call from an ardent, anxious and longing devotee.

The prima-facie view must appreciate the recognition of infinite and intense compassion of God depicted in the *Yoga-Darśana*. Holding God as the Goal as well as means to reach the Goal is the greatest honour only unique to the Lord. The Lord Himself declares:

gatirbhartā prabhuḥ sakṣī nivāsaḥ śaraṇam suhṛt I (B.G. IX-18)

"I am the Supreme Goal, Supporter, Witness, Abode, Refuge and Selfless Friend."

pitāhamasya jagato mātā dhātā pitāmaḥ I (B.G. IX-17)

"I am the Sustainer, and Ruler of this Universe, Its father, mother and grandfather too."

Therefore, Patanjalas honour and not relegate God, as the prima facie view holds, by treating him as what they call a path cleaner pilot and the obliterator of all shackles and obstacles. To answer their doubts we need to put forth the *Gītā* quotation. Let them answer whether or not God is the obliterator of all evils and obstacles or not. Lord Krishna says :

ahṁ tā sarva pāpebhyo mokṣayiṣyāmi mā śucaḥ I (B.G. XVIII-66)

"I shall absolve you of all sins; grieve not"

Ishwara for Patanjalas, is indeed the Goal as well as means to reach that Goal.

Nevertheless omnipotence and inequitable compassion of *Ishwara* lies in His becoming the Reliever and Goal as well. *Ishwara* protects the devotee of His own accord as the sole Guardian, like the cat protecting the kitten.

Before we conclude, let us have a bird's-eye view of theistic practices sown in the *yoga-sūtra*. The theistic practice typified in the first chapter (1/23, 1/28) is a trancive practice or trancive worship. The second chapter introduces the theistic practices for developing virtues and restraint from sins. These practices help the neophyte to inculcate deism and virtuous dispositions to finally gain qualification for wisdom (2/32). For a practitioner of higher hierarchy the aphorist mentions the transfiguration of activities and never-waning deism.

We need to be grateful for the spirited attack of prima-facie view for letting us prove that the theism of yoga is no expediency, no formality, no compromise and no convenience but a spontaneous, intrinsic and profuse deism. The *Ishwara praṇidhāna* is not one of the practices of the *yoga sādhaka,* but as Vyasa puts it in his impeccable style in the *Kriyā-yoga sūtra*, (Y.B. 2/1); it is dedication, devotion and complete resignation to God and consecration of every moment and movement. It knows no termination and interruption. So, is there anything short of absolute and profuse deism in the religious practices of yoga?

❑❑❑

8. Cosmology of Yoga

The whole cosmos, which contains infernal worlds, terrestrial worlds, extra terrestrial worlds and astral planes is totally and undividedly (*otaḥprotaḥ*) pervaded by three *guṇa-s* viz. *sattva, raja* and *tama*. Matter (the five gross elements), infra-matter (infra-atomic structure of matter), and supra-matter (cosmic principle of ego, intelligence (*ahaṁkāra-mahat*) compose the Universe and they are intrinsically and extrinsically composed of the three *guṇa-s*. Therefore, the *prakṛti* (triad of *guṇa-s*) is called as primordial substance of the whole sentient and insentient, movable and immovable creation. The Universe is said to be ensuing from this primordial matter. The aphorist declares (Y.S.4/13) "Whatever is manifest or subtle, is of the nature of *guṇa*".

Now, when the underlying principle of the whole universe is a true entity, the effectual nature cannot be anything but true.

Prakṛti, which is the primordial substance, is subject to law of change (*pariṇāma*) and evolves ever-changing phenomenal Universe. Matter is not only what it is, but also what it becomes; and it is a service of particular perishing presentations. *Prakṛti* is a perpetually fleeting flux without stability. Each object is a fugitive and passes over into different states and later states can be even out of connections with the earlier states. The things in the spatial (limited by space) world come and go in quick succession. The events in the temporal order likewise change and vanish. The body is also subject to mobility, metabolism and catabolism. Oneform of energy is transformed into another and the psychic process is a stream of momentary modifications.

At the outset, a student of yoga philosophy must understand that the metaphysics of yoga is the same as that of *Sāṁkhya* philosophy. Accordingly, the cosmological unfoldment is merely a mutation or transmutation of primal substance which is called as *avyakta*, *pradhāna*, *muḷa prakṛti* or *aliṅga* (which means unmanifest and unmarked primordial matter).

Just as the potency and power in a tiny seed of a banyan tree evolves into a gigantic tree, and figuratively almost from nothing the great thing evolves, the universal unfoldment too, is from nothingness, marklessness and unmanifest, to the markedness and manifest.

The seed of cosmos, therefore, is the primordial matter: the unmanifest called *avyakta*. From this, evolves the *mahat*, the great principle or the first principle as the principle of intelligence or the cosmic principle of intelligence. The metaphysics of yoga calls it *liṅgamātra* or *mahat* or *buddhi* etc. Being the first principle, it is the womb of all diverse creation. It is at this phase, that the creation gets a mark (*liṅga*) and attribute. Although it is womb of all diversities, there is no marked diversity in this first leg of creation. From this principle evolves the *ahaṁkāra* or *Asmita* or ego principle or cosmic ego.

Ahaṁkāra is the third principle and it is here that the *sattva, raja* and *tama* begin their roles with interactions. It is here that infra-atomic structure of matter, senses, mind (psyche) and physique is laid for all embodiments in the Universe. Cosmic ego serves as the field, where the plantation of seed of psycho sensory system, and the material system (*bhūtendriya sṛṣṭi*) takes place.

Thereafter, on one hand, evolve the powers of ten senses and the eleventh sense the mind. While, on the other hand, evolve the infra-atomic structure of gross elements called as *pañca tanmātra*. These five are, *śabda, sparśa, rūpa, rasa and gandha* corresponding to infra-atomic structure of elements of ether, air, fire, water and earth.

From this infra-atomic structure evolve, the gross five elements viz. elements of earth, water, air, fire and ether (*pṛthvī, āp, tej, vāyu ākāśa*). The manifest living creation gets an embodiment by combination of these elements. No embodiment whatsoever, in all the three worlds (infernal, terrestrial and extra-terrestrial) is other than these five elements. The whole of the above process has accounted for the 24 principles of *prakṛti*. In order to make the comprehension easy the same may be tabulated as under:

PRIMORDIAL SUBSTANCE (1)

COSMIC INTELLIGENCE (2)

COSMIO EGO (3)

MIND (4)

SENSES (5 TO 14)

SUBTLE ELEMENTS (15 TO 19)

GROSS ELEMENTS (20 TO 24)

The aphorist has subdivided the evolution of 24 principles into four phases. The primordial substance is *aliṅga* (nuomenal

) which is the unmanifest seed of Creation. From this comes the *liṅgamātra* (phenomenal, marked, Great principle). This is the second phase of Creation. In the third phase of Creation, the principles are undifferentiated and unparticularised. Therefore, it is called as *aviśeṣa parva*. It is at this stage, that the infra-atomic structure of Universe is evolved. This phase is followed by particularised phase called *viśeṣa parva* because creation assumes all diversities in this fourth and final phase.

According to the aphorist, Creation takes place in the following manner:

- Nuomenal : unmanifest stage : *aliëga* : unmarked stage
- Phenomenal : *liëga* : marked stage (cosmic intelligence)
- *aviśeṣa parva :* unparticularised stage (infra structure of mind and matter)
- *viśeṣa parva* : particularised stage (sensory element system)

The above division also accounts for twenty-four principles in the following matter.

1) Noumenal phase	:	1 principle
2) Phenomenal phase	:	1 principle
3) Unparticular phase	:	6 principles
4) Particular phase	:	16 principles.

The six principles categorised under the Unparticularised phase (*aviśeṣa parva*) are cosmic ego and infra-atomic structure of elements of earth, water, fire, air and space. The sixteen principles categorised in the particularised phase are the five conative organs, five cognitive organs, the *manas* (mind) and five gross elements viz., *pṛthvī* (element of earth), *āp* (element of water), *tej* (element of fire), *vāyu* (element of air) and *akaśa* (element of space).

The process of dissolution or deluge is reverse of creation where the particularised phase (*viśeṣa parva*) merges into unparticularised phase (*viśeṣa*). This later gets absorbed into phenomenal or marked phase called as *liṅga parva* to only get final absorption into the noumenal stage of *prakṛti* called as *aliṅga parva*.

On the other lines of cause and effect, the nuomenal has no cause but only effect. As it has no cause it is considered to be a permanent principle (*nitya tattva*). But being subject to change or transmutation, it is not immutable (*apariṇāmī*) Therefore, being noumenal and permanent but mutable end of nature of *guṇa-s*, it stands distinctly different from noumenal, permanent but immutable and *guṇa*-transcendent *Puruṣa*, the SELF.

The great principle, the cosmic principle of intelligence, is the effect of the former and cause of the latter. Similar is the case with the principles evolved in the particularised phase (the eleven senses and five elements). They are effects of the former principles but do not produce anything of the class of principles as effects. They account for diverse visible phenomenal creation which is infinite.

The *Sāṁkhya yoga* doctrine holds that the effects potentially exist in the cause and no effect is altogether new.

The diversity in creation is on account of permutations and combinations of elements which manifest after quintiplication *(pāṅcikaraṇaṁ)*.

It is explicit in the Vyasa *bhāṣya* that the gross elements evolve with the combination of all the five subtle elements. The following table explains this aspect.

1) Evolution of element of space by quintiplication :

50% infra-atomic structure of space.

12.5% infra-atomic structure of air.

12.5% infra-atomic structure of fire.

12.5% infra-atomic structure of water

12.5% infra-atomic structure of earth.

2) Evolution of element of air by quintiplication :

50% infra-atomic structure of air.

12.5% infra-atomic structure of space.

12.5% infra-atomic structure of fire.

12.5% infra-atomic structure of water

12.5% infra-atomic structure of earth.

3) Evolution of fire by quintiplication :

50% infra-atomic structure of fire

12.5% infra-atomic structure of space.

12.5% infra-atomic structure of air.

12.5% infra-atomic structure of water

12.5% infra-atomic structure of earth.

4) Evolution of water by quintiplication :

50% infra-atomic structure of water

12.5% infra-atomic structure of air

12.5% infra-atomic structure of space

12.5% infra-atomic structure of earth

12.5% infra-atomic structure of fire.

5) Evolution of earth by quintiplication :

   50% infra-atomic structure of earth

   12.5% infra-atomic structure of space.

   12.5% infra-atomic structure of air.

   12.5% infra-atomic structure of fire.

   12.5% infra-atomic structure of water.

The above combination is called quintiplication *(pāṅcikaraṇaṁ)*.

❑❑❑

9. Teleology of Yoga

One wonders why there is the limitless and timeless Creation around, above and on all the sides! Does this infinite creation stand to serve some purpose? Is there nothing and absolutely nothing wasteful, extravagant and purposeless in this prolific endless Creation of the Almighty? The feeble intelligence sometimes suggests and sometimes feels for sure, that Creation also consists of useless matter and purposeless things. It also feels that the universe too, is like a commercial and trading market, where there is a dearth of what is wanted and profusion of what is not wanted!

This is a travesty of reality. Teleology comes to prove that the whole, the total and the entire Creation stands for a purpose. Also, not only any purpose but purpose with finality in view which is *bhoga - apavarga*. Every atom, molecule, and corpuscular particle (*aṇureṇū*) stands for that end.

The infinite creation of the Infinite Creator is for Infinite souls. The whole creation is of the nature of *prakṛti*. And it is meant to serve the conscious principle, the *puruṣa*.

The aphorist declares that the very being of creation is for the purpose of *puruṣa* (Y.S.2/21). This *sūtra* along with 2/18, 2/22 articulates teleology of yoga philosophy. The *sūtra-s* convey that all creation which comes to be recognised as a category of knowables, is of the nature of ***sattva, raja*** and ***tama***, consisting of elemental and psycho-sensory substances. The whole creation is for emancipation and experience of ***puruṣa*** (Y.S.2/18). The Creation stands destroyed and sublated for the soul which is emancipated. But the creation physically exists as eternal, because unemancipated souls continue to get served (Y.S.2/22).

The teleology does not only account for purposiveness of Creation but also propounds that, once emancipation is reached and therefore the purpose served, it does not enmesh the soul by remaining as a parasitical plant.

To epitomise this, it may be worded that, yoga-teleology logically and rationally postulates the ***sūtra-s*** 2/18, 2/21, 2/22 :-

a) The whole of Creation, without any exception whatsoever stands and transforms for the purpose of the principle of the class of consciousness having a finality i.e. experience and emancipation in view.

b) The very being of Creation is towards the end mentioned above.

c) With the purpose served totally, Creation does not exist in relation to the respective ***puruṣa***, but continues to remain in the same manner for other souls for whom purposiveness continues.

❑❑❑

10. Ontology of Yoga

Ontology is that branch of metaphysics which ascertains the essential nature of the principles under investigation.

The Universe is visibly diverse containing countless entities from dust to deity. But the metaphysicists of *Sāṁkhya* and yoga have different facts to tell us. The metaphysicists of these systems have declared that there are only two entities in so far as the ultimate reality is concerned. The two entities are absolutely different and distinctly separate.

One reality is the principle of consciousness, the *caitanya tattva* called *puruṣa*, which is permanent, immutable, indestructible, taintless, formless and attributeless conscious principle.

The other principle is the *prakṛti*, the inert matter. The entire Universe is composed of it in the following tiers:

a) Material (elemental: five elements)

b) Infra-material (subtle matter: *tanmātra*)

c) Supra-material (cosmic principle of ego and intelligence)

All these are of the essence of nature of *guṇa*. Therefore the aphorist declares that there be subtle or gross creations and essentially everything is of the nature of *guṇa*. (4/13).

If the question is asked, whether the Almighty has an ontological status or not, the answer is indeed "Yes". Because *Ishwara* of Patanjali *sūtra-s* is not an anthropomorphic concept. The *sūtra-s* defining *Ishwara*, explicitly says that He is the *puruṣa* with distinction. The *sūtra* mentions that *Ishwara* is *puruṣa viśeṣa*. One should not fail to discern that the term *puruṣa* denotes ontological status and nothing short of it. There is a misconception that *Ishwara* of Patanjali *sūtra* refers to personal deity. This is a travesty. The *Ishwara* of the *sūtra* is undoubtedly of the ontological status.

The real concept of *Ishwara* as posited by the *sūtra-s* becomes clear if the textual *sūtra* is kept side by side with hypothetical *sūtra-s* :

Textual *sūtra* is :

kleśa karma vipāka āśayaiḥ aparāmṛṣṭaḥ puruṣaviśeṣaḥ Īśvaraḥ I

Hypothetical *sūtra* would be:

1) *kleśa karma vipāka āśayaiḥ aparāmṛṣṭaḥ Īśvaraḥ I*

2) *kleśa karma vipāka āśayaiḥ aparāmṛṣṭaḥ devatāviśeṣaḥ Īśvaraḥ I*

The hypothetical

sūtra 1 - would have kept *Ishwara* away from ontological status and

sūtra 2 - would have explicitly referred to some personal deity.

Therefore, the term '*puruṣa*' upholds the position that *Ishwara* is of the ontological status and the composite term *puruṣa viśeṣa* mentions that, *Ishwara* is the immanent and transcendental principle which befits the Vedic concept of 'Absolute' or 'Brahman'. The aphorist's wording "*puruṣa- viśeṣa*" is based on the postulation of *puruṣa uttama* in *Bhagavad Gītā*.

In short, the *yoga-sūtra* holds that ontologically, *prakṛti* and *puruṣa* are only two principles characterising the conscious and the non-conscious aspects of the Universe, and that, *Ishwara* is not an anthropomorphic concept but a metaphysical concept.

❑❑❑

11. The Consummation of Yoga

Yoga consummates in what is called *kaivalya*. This is commonly understood as isolation. But this is not an acosmic of solipsism in subjectivity (*niṣprapañcikaraṇam*). It is a release from the enmeshing weftage of *guṇa-s*, and in that sense it is isolation. The *puruṣa*, from time without beginning, is ceaselessly in conjunction with *guṇa-s* through embodiments and transmigrations.

Usually *kaivalya* is understood as emancipation or isolation as that is what it primarily results in. Particularly when the spiritual endeavour commences with the earnest desire to get enfranchised from pains, and when the pains are irrevocably terminated. *Kaivalya* is characterised merely as a release from pain. The use of words by the aphorist such as, "principle of consciousness or power of consciousness establishes in its own nature" (*svarūpa pratiṣṭhā*) in the *kaivalya*, one misconceives it, as an acosmic elipsism coming in subjectively in a painless state. But just as light dispels darkness, pain is expelled by the highest beatitude. It will be desirable to analyse the concept of liberation as a state expressly free from any sensation, be it pain or bliss.

The Vedantins upbraid the Patanjalas by supposing that the *kaivalya* of Patanjali is not desirable and is not the highest attainment or summum bonum described by the Upanishads. It is because *kaivalya* does not grant the beatitude that the human cherishes. The *Patanjalas* can reply thus:

Firstly the beatitude must have a characteristic of the nature of absolute sorrowlessness and these two are the two sides of the same coin. Even the Upanishads declare that liberation is a complete enfranchisement from pain and freedom from embodiments (SVE. UP. 1/11). The conception of *Patanjalas* that in liberation, the *puruṣa* abides in its form is not anything different than what Upanishads declares as '*svena rupena abminispadyate* ' in Chandogya Upanishad (8/12/2).

Kaivalya is unequivocal bliss, and this is what the *Patanjalas* posit. This is expressly stated by Vyasa while commenting on *sūtra* (3/18). He quotes a dialogue of Acharya Jaigisavya and Avattya. Acharya Jaigisavya during the dialogue mentions of highest bliss in *kaivalya*.

The *kaivalya* of Patanjali is characterised by :

a) Final deliverance,

b) Release from the contact of *guṇa-s*

c) Complete destruction of pain,

d) Irrevocable disembodiment,

e) The self attaining its own luminosity,

f) Non-return to the mundane world and

g) Consummation of spiritual endeavour.

❑❑❑

12. Ethico-Religious Aspects of Yoga

A system of thought is mere gymnastics of the intellect, a display of skill in dialectism and a battlefield for polemics, if it does not contain the articulation of an ethico-religious system. In the absence of it, the system of thought offers nothing for practice and remains a futile trade in words.

This aspect of *Darśana* underlines the principles to be inculcated for wisdom and accomplishment of spiritual endeavour. These aspects comprises of positive instructions for the *mumukṣu* (seeker of liberation) from the beginning of all human endeavour to the summum bonum.

Ethico-religious principles work as an alchemy of the mind. These principles are concerned with combining mental cohesiveness with physical virtues rather than mere virtuous physical activities with an inner mutiny. This distinguishes genuine virtue from hypocrisy and semblance of sanctimoniousness. These principles are moral and ethical in general, but bear a special significance for the seeker of essential bliss, beatitude and consummation with the Ultimate.

The *yoga-sūtra* as a *darśana* scores over any system of philosophy in the world, as far as balance in high scholastics and practical instructions are concerned. It has not therefore slipped into abstract dialectics and irreconcilable idealism. Most of the philosophies in the world have tended to be mere intellectual gymnastics, offering nothing whatsoever to a neophyte in search of knowledge. As stated earlier, the *Yoga Darśana* offers everything from a raw beginning to a ripe end in seeking knowledge and realising the Goal.

Some of the philosophies have been so materialistic, that religion has become something intolerable for them and therefore they are ashamed to embrace it. Western scholars have felt that morality and ethics are only meant for upliftment of the savages and the uncultured. The modern philosophies have fumbled to the extent of revolting even against moral and ethical principles and are bent upon creating a civilisation of humans akin to beasts or even worse.

There are very few systems of philosophies which have succeeded in narrowing the gap between Philosophy and Religion and *Yoga Darśana* scores a distinction here over all other systems of thought. Let us compare yoga with some other Indian philosophies:

The monism of Shankaracharya has kept the two branches viz. religion and philosophy apart. He spared no effort in establishing an identity between the individual self and the Universal Self. But in matters of religion, Shankaracharya emphasises a difference in worshipper and the worshipped. The devotional hymns of Adishankara have an outpour of Bhakti for which absolute monism is bitterly opposed. Therefore the gap between religion and philosophy of monism has not been absolutely bridged.

The other *Vedānta* of *Vaishnava-s* have helped religion surmount their philosophical tenet. They have moulded and designed their philosophy to suit religion.

Sāṁkhya has without exception relied on philosophy and has relegated the religious aspect to their twin brother - yoga.

Nyāya and *Vaiśeṣika* have linked themselves with yoga on the issues of an ethico-religious nature. The *Vaiśeṣika-s* have commenced the whole investigation from the definition of *dharma*.

Mimāṁsā system has devoted itself entirely to religion, and philosophy plays a secondary role. It is only the yoga system which has perfect blend and complete mutual accord and a balanced outlook on the two i.e. religion and philosophy.

Now let us try to understand what *dharma* is.

Dharma (merit) is not merely ideal in behaviour, the principles of which come to us just like that or on the behest of a pontiff. *Dharma* is that which results in the upliftment and evolution of man to the highest good. The moral and ethical principles of *dharma* are not towards a social idealism by way of bringing about social relationships based on friendliness, compassion and solicitude. *Dharma* is for the Highest Good of one who adheres to it. Nevertheless, it has an invariable and a concomitant effect on society by arousing a feeling of concern for others.

The ethico-religious principles not only raise the sub-human to the human level, but also take the human to the universal and cosmic level of culture. It is a characteristic of this school of Hindu Philosophy to plant the seedling of theistic consciousness and evolve it to its highest acme, the summum bonum.

In *yoga Darśana*, wherever psychological principles and practical aspects are detailed, the aphorist has framed them as ethico-religious principles. The aphorist is magnanimous in moulding a neophyte into the culture and religion of yoga through *yama* (restraints), which are -

1) non-injury - *ahiṁsā*

2) truthfulness - *satya*

3) non-stealing - *asteya*

4) continence - *brahmacarya*

5) non-hoarding - *aparigraha,*

and -

niyama (observances), which are :

1) cleanliness - *śauca*

2) contentment - *santoṣa*

3) austerities - *tapaḥ*

4) seeking wisdom through self-study and - *svādhyāya*

5) theistic inclination in all actions – *Ishwara praṇidhāna*

The ethico-religious system of *yoga-sūtra* is prominent in the following *sūtra-s*:

1/14 : The *abhyāsa* must be done reverentially and persistently over a long period of time, so that it is firmly rooted.

1/20 : Practice of *samādhi* must be characterised by faith in the instructions of the science of yoga, and it must be practised with energy, zeal, memory, trance and discernment.

1/27 : *prāṇava* (*āuṁ*) is the sacred word which connotes *Ishwara*.

1/26 : The *japa* of '*āuṁ*' is the mode of prayer.

1/32 : For prevention of obstacles in yoga, habitualisation to one truth.

1/39 : Placidity of mind is attained by meditating on deity of one's predilection.

2/10: Austerity, study of spiritual books and surrendering of all actions and fruits thereof to God is ***Kriyā-yoga.***

2/28: The eightfold yoga must be religiously practiced for freedom from impurities and upcoming of wisdom.

2/28: Restraints, observances, postures, control of life-force, subtraction, concentration, meditation, and trance make the eight-fold yoga.

2/30: Restraints are: non-injury, veracity, abstinence from theft, continence and non-hoarding.

2/31: They are great vows, when Universalised and limited by life state, space, time and circumstances.

2/32: Observances are: cleanliness, contentment, austerity, study of philosophical and religious books and inculcation of theist consciousness.

2/33: In case, when opponents of ethico-religious principles dominate, these should be countered with contrary habitualisation.

3/51: When celestial deities and damsels extend invitations, a *yogī* should not accept them or develop a megalomania for having refused.

1/6: The actions of a *yogī* are neither vicious nor virtuous or a combination of both.

4/30: Then, the *yogī* is free from afflictions and actions.

The ethico-religious system is meant to ultimately divinise the human. The escalators are laid by *yama* and *niyama*.

In the initial stages, man is to be made faithful to what he stands for. If a human being has to be a true human being, he must not only be tolerable to humanity but conducive to the progress of humanity and the bio-world. It is only by practising non-injury, truthfulness, non-stealing, non-dissipation or non-sensuality and non-possessiveness that he can be considered more than an average member of human society and the bio-world. Man must try and make minimum compromise with the moral-ethical principles in the business of life. Otherwise he weaves a jungle around him. This is because, by unscrupulousness he is inclined towards violence, falsity, stealing, sensuality and hoarding. Thus greed, passion, self-centredness, lust, anger and hatred will increase. These principles of restraint are therefore common to all cultures, civilisations and religions.

But yoga system has not included these principles in their ethico-religious system from such a narrow perspective. It has its own psychological analysis and altogether different psychodynamics behind the adherence of these universal principles. These principles are found anywhere in world civilisations or in global religions. But it is only the yoga system which has raised these to a high level of ethico-religious principles of unsurpassed value and prominence.

Let us take *ahiṁsā* for analysis. This principle of non-injury has been preached to abate the passion, lust, hatred, and anger in a human being. Besides, it helps to spread friendliness, brotherly feeling, and compassion. But is it going to help one to do the highest good i.e.

to attain the highest realisation for release from bondage. Yoga sees in *ahiṁsā* a technique to attain an unagitated state of mind. This absence of agitation creates a mental quietude, which in turn prepares ground for meditation. Meditation brings trance and then an intuitive mystic vision, and finally the highest good. Since *hiṁsā* is invariably an outcome of inner agitation, yoga-psychology strikes the fact that *ahiṁsā* is one side of the coin which has non-agitation as the other side of it.

Non-agitation is followed by quietude, internalisation, meditation, trance and revelation. Therefore the psychodynamics behind a *yogī's ahiṁsā* is not a desire to grant fearlessness to men and creatures around, but he aims at non-agitation and quietude for revelation. Of course the development of qualities of love and fearlessness are a by-product of *ahiṁsā* practice.

Now let us take veracity or truthfulness called *satya*. A *yogī* does not aim at credibility when he practices truthfulness nor granting fearlessness towards others. But his vow of *satya* obtains for him a power through which he can realise all that he wishes. Therefore he is in a position to sublate all that antagonises his inner aim. This vow of truthfulness generates complete convenience to his endeavour. When all his wishes are fulfilled the *yogī* acquires a non-agitated state of mind and then the same chain of desirables leads to revelation by adhering to truth. Therefore a *yogī* aims at a mental state which is conducive to the final objective of freedom.

It will be interesting to note that when a moralist or ethical minded worldly man is obstinate in following this principle of truthfulness, he is more agonised and antagonised by the ways of world. A worldly man will never be at peace by scrupulously following the path of truthfulness. He is fumbled and bruised in the world more than a man who is not moral or ethical minded. His despair, dejection and agony is more. It is because it is an impractical ideal when it is practiced from the point of view of obstinacy. The army of scrupulous morality and ethicality can only prove self agonizing for a man with indiscriminative worldliness. The moralist saddles what the world antagonises. Therefore he is agonised and agitated. But a Yoga Practitioner does not dive into the ocean of the world with these principles aback. He is never an over enthusiastic world-monger.

There is a substantial compendium in his worldliness. He is never extravagant and flamboyant. Therefore, there are less fumblings, less bruises, less agitations and agonies. The restraint aspect from excessive worldliness helps him follow all *yama* principles more scrupulously, and apply the *yogīc* psycho-dynamics more successfully.

Coming to non-stealing, first let us understand what it is. It is an absence of objective desire and thirst for objects. When one is aware of the eternal glory and grandeur of the self, the thirst and passion wanes too and finally gets destroyed. It is in vain to preach non-stealing to a destitute. But when glory of the soul is tasted there can be no psycho-dynamics for stealing. Therefore by the practice of non-stealing what is implied is that a yoga practitioner must be in search of inner glory, so that he may loose the thirst and acquire a non-agitative state of mind leading to meditation and trance for philosophical revelation.

Celibacy too has quite a different connotation in yoga. It is not practised with a view to develop mastery over sexual instinct. The dissipation is bound to follow on account of inner turbulence, infatuation and blind instinct. This infatuation is the result of excessive darkness of *tamas*. Just as the sun can be eclipsed by a tiny moon, virtue, intelligence and discrimination can be eclipsed by a spot of *tamas* or infatuation. It can make or cause even an enlightened one to falter. Since *tamas* is a foe of *sattva* and since *sattva* is the material cause of *samādhi*, a yoga practitioner takes up celibacy with these psycho-dynamics. He is wary of dissipation because it leads to dominance of *tamas* which eclipses *sattva*. This nullifies all search for the final beatitude and freedom. Therefore a yoga practitioner's pursuit of celibacy is not for moral or ethical reasons only or to win a credibility and appreciation or confidence of control over the opposite sex..

Non-hoarding called *aparigraha* has the same reason as the one given for celibacy. It is based on non-possessiveness which brings desirelessness, which in turn takes a Sadhaka to higher pursuits.

Now let us analyse the second limb of *Aṣṭāṅga yoga* called *niyama*. The *niyama* are cleanliness, contentment, austerities, self-study, and dedication and devotion to the Lord.

The cleanliness called *śauca* that is practised by a *yogī* is not with a view to good hygiene or cosmetics. For him, cleanliness is inseparable from purity, chastity and guilelessness. Cleanliness, chastity and guilelessness account for quietude, peace and tranquility of mind. One can now easily trace the *yogī's* quality of cleanliness and chastity. The tranquility of mind, so earned can amount to restraint in the mind and meditation/trance-revelation.

Patanjali is quite explicit on the point stated above when he speaks of internal cleansing. In the aphorism which says : "And upon the essence becoming pure, come high mindedness, one pointedness, control of the senses and fitness for knowledge of the soul (2/14)". It is evident here that cleanliness is not merely a code of ethics or morality or hygiene but it is an aspect of ethico-religious system. Needless to add that the physical hygiene automatically follows spiritual cleansing.

Contentment is the second *niyama*. The moralist and ethical minded people adore it because lack of it amounts to agitation, despair, anger, hatred etc. More often than not the contentment practised by a moralist is only a semblance of it. It is in fact an outcome of defeatism. Such contentment is actually antagonistic to yoga-psychology. Because a show of contentment or contentment born of helplessness or defeat contain tremendous inner violence and turbulence. Desires, needs and aspirations are under tremendous pressure which lead to violence.

But the contentment of a yoga practitioner is evolved out of quite a different psychodynamics. It is never composed of blocks of helplessness or defeat or failure. It is an outcome of loss of or waning of the very thirst for the worldly things in preference to the higher principles.

Just as a student under the fever of exams finds the cupid tendencies waning although he is in the prime age of youth, the yoga practitioner is ever concerned with the highest goal, which is Self-realisation. It is therefore that in preference to the highest the passion for lower mundane things wane. The yoga practitioner is face to face with the great glory within. He practices it for mental quietude, solace, and passivity to proceed towards meditation, trance and revelation. With contentment, the tumult, uproar, and bustle of worldly life come to an end. The moderation and simplicity that the contentment brings in one's life, makes the *yogī*'s life worthy of *yogīc* pursuits.

Tapa is the third *niyama* inadequately translated as austerities. There is no English term for *tapa*. Let us see what *tapa* is. The very word is etymologically associated with heat. Heat as a form of energy has proved its capacity in "Thermo-dynamics" of Physics. The very act of *tapa* is to work the thermodynamics within the physic-mental system and bring forth desired fruit. Therefore *tapas* is not merely mortification or indiscrete rigidity. It is not a mere energy generation required for a particular end in life. It is energy generation, allocation and management.

The spiritual path is an upward climb and an avoidance of downward sliding. To tread upwards one requires higher power-allocation of energy. It is *tapas* which engenders it. The avoidance of the downward slide is attained by going in deep friction with natural movement. Here too, because of friction, heat is generated. Therefore, *tapas* is a sort of bio-psycho-religious thermodynamics to climb upward on the spiritual path and avoid a downward glide to oblivion.

So *tapa* is not a meaningless rigidity and excessive control but a discrete generation and release of power.

Another peculiarity of *tapa* is that it is a major component of all the practical aspects of yoga. Without the help of *tapa* one cannot move from *hiṁsā* to *ahiṁsā*, *asatya* to *satya, steya* to *asteya*, *abrahmacharya* to *brahmacarya*, *parigraha* to *aparigraha*, *aśauca* to *śauca*, *asantoṣa* to *santoṣa*, *asvādhyāya* to *svādhyāya* and *anīśvara praṇidhāna* to *Ishwara praṇidhāna*. Similarly from absence of *āsana* practice to practice of *āsana* and *prāṇāyāma* etc.

The main feature of a *yogic tapa* is to lessen the thirst and hunger of the body and lessen the pleasures of the senses, so that quietude sets in and higher psychological practices of yoga can be made possible.

Svādhyāya is the fourth *niyama* which is primarily of the nature of study of philosophical aspects of life and promotion of religious approach to life. By *svādhyāya*, the yoga practices are done with understanding and discernment rather than mechanically. '*Japa*' is another aspect of *svādhyāya*, in its technical sense, it is a way for the worship of the extra-terrestrial deities. This helps one win their grace and smoothen the path. It also directly helps in converging the mental forces to a very mental act. *Japa* is one of the major ways which leads towards meditation.

Ishwara praṇidhāna means "all in all". It is one and only way for all ends. In the path of spiritualism it is a means as well as an end. The very purpose of devotion and worship of God, in all faith, is peace and tranquility of mind.

Therefore, there need be no use of words to explain the role of *Ishwara praṇidhāna* in yoga.

This speaks of the importance that author has accorded to the ethico-religious principles. It is on this account of unreserved acceptance and incorporation of practical aspect in its philosophy that the yoga system has served as a philosopher's stone (*parīsa*) to the other Indian philosophies irrespective of their being orthodox or heterodox.

❑❑❑

13. Mysticism and Intuitive Mysticism of Yoga

By mysticism what is to be understood here is not just the spiritual occultism, but the mysteries of all sciences, philosophies and life. All that goes beyond the analytical faculty of human intelligence and comes within the grasp of intuitive faculty of human intelligence is termed here as mysticism. The intuitive mysticism is the *yogīc* process of envisionment.

Advancement in any branch of knowledge is always and invariably marked by a trace of mysticism in its theories and dictums. The abstract aspect in the finer phase or more advanced stage of all universal physical phenomena has startled even the scientists of high calibre. It might be true that mysticism is inevitable in any field of study when an advanced stage is reached.

Towards the end of this century, physics, the base of all modern knowledge, has come to discern a cloud of mysticism hanging over it. Soon the world will crawl into metaphysics from physics, which will mark a new era in the development of human intelligence. The world of scientific intellectuals has come to realise that what lies in the realm of physics is too insignificant of part of the Universal phenomenalism. And what lies beyond physics is truly warped by an enigmatic cloud of mysticism. Since metaphysics is full of mysticism, scientists will not be able to extricate themselves from enigma with the help of intellectual rationalism and empirical positivism that has served them all along.

Mysticism has been for some reasons closely associated with occultism. But it is only recently that physicists have come out with a declaration of what they call "Mysteries of Physics". This development of physics in the west truly testifies to the veracity of eastern or oriental intelligence. This element of mystery can now be traced in all branches of knowledge. Let's take an example of mystery in physics. If a fifty year old astronaut travels in space at the velocity of light of fifty years and comes back to earth, he might find his son older than him physically and mentally by many years, thus making the father far younger than the son. This is because, according to the physicists, the space traveller voyaging at the velocity of light transcends the concept of time and hence does not age during the course of his journey.

We come across many such enigmatic, mystical and abstruse dogmas, dictums and theories in the field of '*Darśana*' (Indian Philosophical System), because they deal with metaphysical aspects of Universe and '*Dharma*' is commonly understood as religion. Since *Darśana* establishes a base for the knowledge of subtle matter and infra-matter elements in the Universe and beyond, it is replete with mysteries, obscurities, enigmas and conundrums to only confuse human intelligence which has an apathy for any mode of knowledge other than empirical rationalism.

Since the analytical process of intelligence ultimately gives way to mysticism, this process of knowledge is monopolised by a handful of great scientists who have the spark of intuition. Those who have super vision and super normal faculty of intuition like Einstein lead the way. It seems that capacity for intuition is regulated by chance. But intuitive mysticism is the womb for intuitive faculty. And the intuitive mysticism of yoga has developed this process for evolution of this rare and highly sought after faculty.

In the science of spiritualism called '*Adhyātma*' intuitive mysticism is understood, by even a common man, as '*Divyacakṣu*' or '*Divya dṛṣṭi*'. In the *Gītā*, the cosmic form of Lord Krishna is said to have been envisioned by Arjuna with *divya cakṣu* (Chapter 11). The projected cosmic form of Lord Krishna beheld by Arjuna was not a miracle performed by Lord Krishna nor did he bewitch Arjuna with a spell of hallucination. The vision was absolutely real and the vision of cosmic form of Lord Krishna was also equally real. Arjuna describes the mystery as 'endless without beginning and endless end with no centre as middle point', for the form of Krishna - the Cosmic being. Arjuna for the first time beheld Krishna in His essential, true and real form, the timeless form. But that vision was not granted to all those thousands who had gathered around Arjuna to battle. Since, the vision was only for Arjuna, of course with few exceptions of super-humans, it was an envisionment of the nature of intuitive mysticism - a *yogī*c power of envisionment which was granted by Krishna to Arjuna alone. Here, the mystery was in Krishna's true form as Cosmic Being and Infinite Being. The process through which Arjuna got the vision was intuitive mysticism. This passage intends to bring out the mysticism in the Religion and Philosophy of yoga and understand the process to unravel the enigmas by their vision through valid intuitions outlined in the practical aspects of yoga.

The mystical aspect of yoga Philosophy is concerned with theorising the Universal phenomenalism for Creation and define the nuomenal- the subject matter of metaphysics.

The definition of metaphysical entities like soul and unmanifest primal substance of Universe and the description of Universe in its rudimentary stages form the mysticism of yoga Philosophy. The mysticism of religion of yoga lies in its mention of *yogīc* powers to penetrate subtle, veiled and hidden matter, and the theism of yoga and science of Karma outlined in the system.

In intuitive mysticism of yoga, we try to understand how a *yogī* gets knowledge of subtle-matter, infra-matter and supra-matter with such ease as though this knowledge was at his fingertips. It is here we shall try to understand the process of spontaneous intuitive flash, which helps reveal the subtle world. The theory of intuitive knowledge process has been spelt out in the *yoga-sūtra-s*. This theory is quite ambiguous for human intelligence to grasp. Therefore the analysis of this process will be presented here. The yoga system in its practical aspects has outlined the process by which this faculty can be awakened and evolved. The same will be explained in this passage.

This intuitive mysticism is a sudden spark. It is a spontaneous and instantaneous lightening sparkle that illuminates the human intelligence, as well as an object of knowledge, psychologically and simultaneously. Therefore, it has been radically understood as an intuitive flash. It almost seems self-generated and self-born and an independent psycho-intellectual phenomenon.

This intuitive mysticism is the acme of all knowledge in that aspect of revelation. No knowledge can ever be finer or score over it. The derivation, and theorisation monitored in intuitive mysticism are irrefutable, interminable and irrevocable anywhere at any time. Since knowledge becomes final and absolutely comprehensive by intuitive mysticism, there need not be and there can be no further pursuit of knowledge. As a matter of fact, the entire spiritual endeavour of human being comes to an end at this stage. Since spiritual science aims at bequeathing summum bonum to the way-farer on the path of spiritualism, yoga as a complete science of human being has accomplished a very deep, complete and comprehensive reflection on this subject. As a matter of fact this branch of yoga system called 'Intuitive Mysticism', forms an important limb of yoga system.

All knowledge begins from sensory knowledge, sensations and thought process in the brain. Psychology of perception and physiology of perception completes this process. Direct perception, inference, the testimonial evidence from authoritative books of science and expert guidance of teachers, complement this knowledge process.

But when the subject of knowledge pertains to meta-physics, religion and spiritualism, knowledge process begins not with sensory perception or sensation, but it begins with the teachings of Vedic sciences. The whole knowledge process here, is based on postulations and instructions found in the revelations (Veda) and traditional texts (*smṛti and śṛti*). Therefore, the root of all metaphysical, religious and spiritual knowledge is in our ancient sciences in general and Veda in particular, which the Cosmic Being has granted us at the beginning of Creations in all Cosmic cycles. The fruit of knowledge or culmination of knowledge process is in intuitive mysticism. In short, the root of all higher knowledge is the instructions of ancient ***śāstra-s*** and revered *ācārya-s*, while the fruit of culmination of all knowledge is in intuitive mysticism.

In the first stage the seeker on the spiritual path, very beseechingly and humbly takes the first gift of knowledge from the ***Ācārya*** or from the holy books. In the second stage, the seeker effects what is called as 'Internal spray'. Here he uses the intellectual process, analytical process and logical process without the slightest doubt in the postulates of ancient sciences, cultures and knowledge gained in the first stage. Therefore, the instructions coming from the sciences or preceptors may be considered as external spray while the logical reasoning, analytical process maybe considered as an internal spray. The internal spray helps to correct and deepen the impressions of knowledge gained in the first stage. The completion of internal spray qualifies the seeker for the second stage of instructions at a comparatively advanced stage. The second stage of study and instructions feeds the intellect and enhances its capacity for more cogent reasoning and analysis and intellectual processing. Therefore, the two processes complement each other and make the study more penetrating and analytical reasoning more exact and precise. This is how a strong and comprehensive structure of knowledge is raised. Does this chain process ever culminate in finality of knowledge? No, never. The finality of knowledge is only in intuitive mysticism. Knowledge process culminates here because the knowledge in intuitive mysticism is a vision of the nature of its essence and the knowledge is all-dimensional.

Before finding the link between the first two phases of knowledge (described as external spray and internal spray, which are the seed and sprout of knowledge) and the culminating phase of intuitive mysticism (the final fruit), let us compare the intuitions that we commoners experience and the intuitive mysticism of a *yogī*.

One is familiar with sudden, spasmodic and unexpected flash perception or internal perception which we term as intuition. This intuition and intuition now under discussion called as intuitive mysticism are poles apart. Mistaking the two as one, would be a grave error. The intuition experienced by the uninitiate commoners is an intellectual implosion. The knowledge which is consciously processed in the brain suddenly and unexpectedly projects itself on the intellectual screen. These are in fact effects of an accidental convulsion in the psycho-cerebral system.

But in the intuitive mysticism the process of study/instruction and reflection continues over a long time. The seeker is also invariably a highly advanced practitioner of *Aṣṭāṅga yoga*. This intuitive mysticism is only an outcome of practice of trance. Therefore unless the practice of trance has been experienced intuitive mysticism cannot be realised. The psyche must have exuberance of *samādhi* potentials. The *samādhi* impressions created by constant practice of integrated *Aṣṭāṅga yoga* in general and *samādhi* in particular, cleanse the psyche and make it a pure virgin womb for pure conception and spontaneous deliverance of knowledge. An important feature of intuitive mysticism is that it always comes forth in a subjective state of internalisation. Therefore, the intuition devoid of trancive practice and therefore devoid of *samādhi* impressions, is faulty, lopsided and imperfect as well as accidental.

However, the flash that a *yogī* begets would range from minimum fault to maximum precision and perfections. The provision of fault and flaw is on account of incomplete persuasion in the practical aspects of yoga and non-attainment of higher levels in the hierarchy of yoga. This has been made clear to emphasise the fact that there are various levels of hierarchy in all aspects of practical yoga and that all the intuitions of yoga practitioners need not be considered faultless, whatever be the nature of these intuitions or intuitive experiences.

Now all the issues which come under the realm of metaphysics cannot be subjected to empirical reasoning, the reasoning and logical process based on sensory perception. The various intellectual analysis opted by intellectual rationalism are :

1) Conceptual analysis

2) Definitive analysis

3) Propositive analysis

4) Synthetical analysis

while the various logical processes are :

1) Inductive logic

2) Deductive logic

3) Logic of chance

4) Logic of Philosophy.

These cannot serve in metaphysics as they serve in all other fields of knowledge. What one wants to clarify here is, that the metaphysical entities like soul and God cannot be found and discerned with these mortal eyes and temporal intelligence. Howsoever the scientist may scramble and bustle round the world and above in the limitless space in search of God, with microscope and telescopes, all that will be in vain. Although He exists in every single atomic particle and pervades the Universe and Beyond, *Upanişadic* sageaptly says :

"It moves and it moves not;

It is far and it is near;

It is within all this;

And also outside all this"

(ISA U.P.5)

Let that be as it may. Despite the fact that God cannot be revealed by subjecting it to logic, empiricism and intellectualism, the Buddhist's atheistic and anti-soul dialectics were successfully answered by the orthodox Logician Jñānācārya. The arguments of the *Ācārya* were just well put in his marvellous *Nyāyakusumāñjali.* The Buddhists had strong antipathy towards Vedic teachings. Therefore they could be convinced only by Logic, verbal squabble and intellectual gymnastics. The *Ācārya* truly succeeded in his mission.

But the fact remains, that soul and God can only be understood by intuitive mysticism termed as *'gūḍha sākṣātkāra'* --- nevertheless the instructions of the Vedas and instructions coming from Vedic *ācārya-s* lay the foundation for it. In this context, it will be worth noticing that testimonial cognition (scriptures) scores over direct perception and inference. Also, the logical process, analytical process and intellectual process which are coherent with scriptures, contribute substantially compared to none by direct and indirect perception. Therefore, instructions of Vedic sciences and instructions from Vedic

Gurus sow the seed of wisdom, and intuitive mysticism is the fruit. This vision is a visualisation of Vedic verbal theories. The intellectual and analytical process form the whole tree and thus serve as indispensable mediators. The whole process of knowledge here unifies all the scriptural postulates, intellectual processing and mystic vision.

Therefore our ancient academies in the spiritual sciences called *adhyātma* had the following injunctions:

1) Beseechingly and reverentially receive the instructions from teachers and sciences.

2) Subject the knowledge so gained, with constant deliberations, ponderings and reflections, through logical process and analytical process to properly amend and deepen the impressions.

3) Take a rereading or repeated instructions and reprocessing by internal methods of reflections and analysis to cultivate the impressions gained through knowledge. And cyclically repeat the process by deeper instructions and deeper reflections.

4) Meanwhile continue with the practice of yoga for cleansing the psyche and attain meditation, single pointedness and introcessed meditations. Develop the capacity for higher psychological practices of yoga (*samādhi*)

5) And patiently wait for the incredible intuitive flash in an internalised state of mind.

At this stage, one is sorely tempted to compare the modern academical method of pursuit of the esoteric of modern sciences with the ancient method of savant sages who imparted spiritual sciences. The modern method which has spread over the entire globe is based on intellectual rationalism.

The thinkers, philosophers, and scientists have held high esteem in the method. All other approaches are subject to this autocratic and dictatorial court of intellectual rationalism for evaluation and scrutiny. There was an era where blind faith chaired the court and ruthlessly stamped the intellectualism and positivism with blind fury. That was one extreme of obstinacy. Now, autocracy of intellectual rationalism has reached the other end of obstinacy to impede the development of human evolution. Granting of irrefutable validity and unquestionable acceptance to intellectual rationalism will lead to the insolvency of human intelligence in times ahead. It is now high time we realised that intellectual rationalism has its own limits and that these limits terminate well before knowledge reaches its zenith. Scientists after Einstein have heralded these limitations of intellectual rationalism though still in largely muffled voices.

They have come to accept something like the mysteries of Physics. Physics in the past few decades has made incredible strides and has come to discover the realm of metaphysics to which they give the epithet 'Mysteries', because scientists have encountered some dualities and contradictions which cannot be explained away by intellectual rationalism. Their analyses have been paralysed and intelligence has been benumbed by the enigmas of higher physics such as astrophysics and particle physics. An example may convince the reader that intellectual process has an end before knowledge can culminate and it will not be too long before we hoist the white flag of intellectualism. As a branch of advance physics has arrived at the conclusion that energy moves in particles and at the same time it has also accepted the theory that energy moves in waves. This contradiction poses a problem for the elite class of scientists. Hence these scientists have resorted to mutterings - "Mysteries of Physics". This in a way is like issuing a white paper on intellectual rationalism.

This should not lead one to look down upon intellectual rationalism. Because in all fields of knowledge, except metaphysics, religion and spiritualism, it has its indisputable importance. But what is aimed at, in the above example is the realisation of acceptance of process which transcends empirical knowledge and which is intuitive mysticism. Secondly, that in the pursuit of higher sciences like metaphysics, the *yogīc* process of internal cleansing debilitates the knowledge eclipsing factors and obliterates all impressions and memories that arise on account of subconscious tendencies. The religion of yoga bestows faultless creative intelligence which is the main source of the higher fields of knowledge.

It is also worthwhile to note that scientists from Archimedes to Newton and then down to Einstein, came out with their ecstatic research. Their epoch-making discoveries were not out of test-tube observations or laboratory experiments. It was the incredible intuitive flash which was quite ecstatic, that put them in the forefront of the scientific world. At this point it is desirable to point out that one does not discount the logical conclusions, mathematical derivations, statistical derivations and rationale based on logical reasoning, intellectual rationalism and scientific process of empirical positivism. The intellectual process has been duly recognised in the epistemology of yoga when the stage of intellectual analysis and logical analysis were included in the knowledge process. Indian philosophers in general and Patanjalas in particular, were never reluctant to embrace the logical process, analytical process, and intellectual process. As a matter of fact among the scholastics of Indian philosophy, the logical approach and empirical study can be traced in abundance. The Indian logicians headed by sage Gautama were the pioneers of the intellectual process. Nowhere in the world was the flag of intellectual rationalism hoisted before the Indian classical logicians. But since the Indian system of logic and intellectual rationalism was founded by sages and seers, there was no element of extreme obstinacy behind their clinging to the intellectual process. It is interesting to study how they outlined the process of knowledge. The aphorisms of Gautama begin with an exhaustive aphorism. Indian classical logic or Indian Realism as it is called was a *darśana* and therefore the *sūtra*:-

Pramāṇa prameya saṁśaya prayojana dṛṣṭānta
siddhāntāvayava tarkanirṇaya vādajalpa
vitaṇḍāhetvābhāsacchalajātinigraha sthānānām
tattvajñānānniśreyasādhigamaḥ I (N.S. 1.1.1)

"Supreme felicity is attained by the knowledge about true nature of sixteen categories, viz.,

- Means of knowledge,
- Object of right knowledge,
- Doubt,
- Purpose,
- Familiar instances,
- Established tenets,
- Members of tenets, (constituents of tenets)
- Confutation/Hypothetical reasoning,
- Ascertainment,
- Discussion,

- Wrangling (Honest Wrangling)
- Purposeful cavil,
- Fallacy,
- Quibble,
- Futility, and
- Occasion for rebuke.

Wrangling and quibbling etc., were included for the fact that the intellectual substance could be cultured for knowledge. It is evident here that Indian logicians held high the path of intellectual rationalism. But since the founders of that system were seers and sages, they did not fail to realise the limitations of intellectual process. They finally conceded the culmination of knowledge to *samādhi* of yoga, which is but intuitive mysticism.

The aphorist of that system says:

(*samādhi viśeṣa abhyāsāt*) (N.S. 4.2.36)

i.e. acceptance of the fact that culmination of knowledge is in the womb of the practice of *samādhi*. Therefore he outlines *Aṣṭāṅga yoga*.

Intellectual rationalism no doubt may fathom reality and its processes and may infer the nature of reality by deductive process. But all its derivations will be in stages and compartments. But the conclusion reached by an intuitive mystic is all at one stroke. The ecstatic flash does transgress the logical stage of analysis, but its derivations are never illogical. It is because, before the ecstatic and mystical flash, the mystic has already gone through the logical process, analytical process and scientific process.

However immaculate, faultless and flawless intellectual rationalism may be and however ripe it may be, it will only and in humbly offering obeisance to the Infinite Universal Principle, at the gates of Shrine only. While, the mystic will reach the sanctum sanctorum of the shrine and will merge in the Infinite. That will be the end of all spiritual endeavor.

The revelations of a *yogī* are immediate, direct and spontaneous while that of the intellectual rationalist, indirect and mediate.

This culminative knowledge process is tripartite.

1) Direct perception, scriptural and tutorial instructions.

2) The internal processing of knowledge by logical process, analytical process and intellectual process.

3) The practice of yoga principles, cleansing the psyche developing the capacities for *yogīc* concentration and meditation-qualifying for ecstatic intuitive spark and intuitive mysticism.

Now a question can be asked as to where this tripartite knowledge process has been enunciated in the *yoga-sūtra-s* of Patanjali. Of course since the whole text of *yoga-sūtra* is so very brief and pithy, the above purport is to be traced in the implicit aspect of the science. Besides, a descriptive process has no place in aphoristic texts. Therefore a detailed investigation cannot be expected from the aphorist or the commentators. Moreover, since we have deprived ourselves of traditional academies, much has become obscure.

Let us try to understand the above mentioned issue, through the implicit content of yoga System. In the second chapter of *yoga-sūtra-s*, the aphorist sums up the whole investigation of intuitive mysticism in just two aphorisms. In the twenty sixth aphorism on liberation which is the summum bonum of all human endeavour, the aphorist says that undisturbed discriminative discernment is the means for the attainment of the highest. He uses the word *'khyāti'* for discernment in preference to *jñāna*. The terms knowledge and discernments are to be understood with all distinctions. If *'khyāti'* is to be translated as discernment, one must specify its meaning to suit the fundamental purport here. Let us therefore compare it with the term 'Knowledge' to distinguish it from the same. Knowledge (*jñāna*) indicates the knowing aspect of a fact or an object. It may be a conclusion arrived at, by logical process, analytical process or mathematical process. It may not necessarily be revelation. But discernment (*khyāti*) must be invariably taken as revelation in this context, and not the conclusion arrived at by intellectual or scientific processes.

Now what is to be discerned in the current aphorism is discriminative discernment. This is an actual envisionment of difference in the nuomenal primordial matter and nuomenal soul. The envisionment of nuomenal entities cannot occur through sensory vision or empirical process. Therefore it must be understood that what is suggested here is a vision coming from intuitive mysticism. If the aphorist had used the term *jñāna* (knowledge) instead of *khyāti* (discernment), the whole concept of intuitive mysticism could not have been even forcibly interpolated or even imagined in this system of thought. This is a stark example of subterranean import that most of the *yoga-sūtra-s* have.

In short, an envisionment of nuomenal entity can occur only by the mystic vision, ecstatic mystic flash or intuitive mysticism, all being of one and the same category. All these are visions that come in a trance or a state of subjectivistic introcession. Therefore, we arrive at another characteristic of it, that intuitive mysticism is the outcome of a state of trance, which is exclusively a deep introcession.

Secondly, this discernment has to be absolutely flawless, immaculate, perfect and complete. This has been immediately made explicit by the aphorist in the twenty seventh *sūtra*. This particular feature of it sets it apart from the common man's intuition or an ecstatic spark of insight. The aphorist says that in this culminative knowledge, there are seven envisionments each being absolutely final, complete and total.

Therefore the implicit and explicit purport of the two *sūtra-s* 26 and 27 heave the towering subject matter of intuitive mysticism. A sincere student of *yoga-sūtra* must ponder over these terms in these two *sūtra-s*. He must investigate as to why the aphorist has opted for the term *'khyāti'* in preference to *jñāna*. Another point of investigation is the mention of uninterrupted envisionment or irrevocable vision of finality which of course is to accentuate the summum bonum or and of all spiritual endeavour. Finally, with what purport in mind does the aphorist explicitly mention that the seven envisionments must be final and ultimate?

Now let us trace the tripartite process of intuitive mysticism suggested in the aphorism either explicitly or by implicit instructions. The first stage of receiving instructions from a preceptor or from scriptures may be traced in '*svādhyāya*' of '*niyama*' and *'Kriyā yoga'*. Vyasa, the commentator explicitly mentions that it is a study of spiritual books. And the study called Adhyatma implies the intellectual process, the logical process, the reflective process, the analytical process

This leads us to the second stage of 'internal spray' as detailed earlier. The *Aṣṭāṅga yoga* is recommended for destroying the impurities in the mind and resultant brightening of the flame of knowledge until the ultimate objective of knowledge is attained (Y.S.2/28). Therefore, we may observe that the subject matter of intuitive mysticism is dealt with in the *sūtra-s* of *Kriyā yoga niyama* (*svādhyāya*), *Aṣṭāṅga yoga* (2/28) and the 26th, and 27th *sūtra-s* of the second chapter.

The student of philosophy or seeker of knowledge must know for sure that there is no alternative to intuitive mysticism if the ultimate culmination of knowledge is to be attained for any branch of knowledge from Physics to Meta-Physics. If perfection in that branch of knowledge is to be attained, there must be faultlessness, non-contortions and non-distortions in the psyche. That will develop meditative faculties and bestow qualification for intuitive mysticism. Integrated practice of *Aṣṭāṅga yoga* is truly indispensable for the attainment of higher knowledge.

A critique may pose some questions here:-

Does the theorist here mean to say that Archimedes, Newton and Einstein and other great scientists and thinkers practised this *Aṣṭāṅga yoga* or did they attain the capacity for immaculate spark without *Aṣṭāṅga yoga*? Let us answer these questions. There should be no doubt that they had extraordinary concentrative and reflective faculties, and a steady, non-spasmodic mind and intelligence. They had their mind internally cleansed. The austerities that are required to cleanse the psyche must have been observed in previous lives, because there has to be a cause for effect. It should be interesting here to note that what we have considered super brain for geniuses like Einstein was not really because of the structure of the brain, which encased some extra or special neurons in the brain, but were geniuses by birth. Because when his brain was dissected after death, they found no difference in the geography, physics and physiology of his brain from the brain of a common man. Therefore, from the oriental point of view, the extraordinary feats that Einstein's intelligence produced was not the result of the structure of the brain in the skull, but a culmination of his previous births. And that infra-brain had laid the foundation for the brain of Einstein. Therefore, Einstein had evolved over many, many previous lives before he became the incredible Dr. Einstein!

This intuitive mysticism has an uncommon place in metaphysics because the issues that pertain to metaphysics are:

1) Infra-atomic particles of gross matter (something like subatomic particles of particle-physics)

2) Cosmic ego

3) Cosmic intelligence

4) Primal substance

5) Soul or the spirit

6) Divinity or the Absolute.

It is evident that these matters are beyond sensory, intellectual and mathematical process for realisation because the above processes may only make us to infer those.

The finer aspect of religion, in the sense, the oriental mind understands *dharma*, has be investigated not by intellectual processes or any mortal authority on *dharma*. But it has to be accepted in one's own heart provided it has been raised to an exalted state. *Mahābhārata* very correctly says that the principle of *dharma* (concept of vice and virtue) is deep down in the heart, very much obscured. The *dharma* in the oriental sense cannot be examined outside one's heart of conscience.

Therefore one must do a deep search well beneath the subliminal impressions and reach the heart, and examine what is right and wrong for one's self. Of course, we ordinary mortals have no qualifications or authority to examine our *dharma*. We must abide by books on *dharma* and the commandments of *Paṇdita-s* of *dharma*.

Let us take an example to illustrate how misleading it would be to define or explain our *dharma* by the process of logical analysis or a rational intellectual approach. Let us compare the two episodes-one from the Ramayana and the other from the *Mahābhārata*. Bhishma was a great devotee of the Lord who was the hero of *Mahābhārata*. Vibhishana was a devotee of equal acclaim in the Ramayana. But both the devotees acted in opposition to one another though under similar and identical situations. But both were right from the point of view of *dharma*. Bhishma fought the great battle leading the non-righteous army and he fought against the beloved Lord, because he did not wish to betray those who were his dependents. While Vibhishana who was his equal as a devotee of the Lord betrayed his elder brother Ravana and fought against the non-righteous, and fought for the Lord.

Now let us analyse the facts:

Bhishma fought against his Lord as it was his *dharma* not to betray those who depended on him and fought for the unrighteous people against the righteous people.

Vibhishana fought in association with his Lord betraying his brother who depended on him and fought for the righteous people against the unrighteous people. Here, both the subjects were righteous devotees of the Lord and were of equal status. But they acted contrarily. Now, if this episode is sought to be understood by the logical and analytical method, under the banner of intellectual rationalism, one can never reconcile with the reality that both were right, correct and faultless. But the supreme court of *dharma* acquitted them of any charge and declared them not only faultless but proclaimed them as meritorious. The judgement too was faultless. What is this enigma? The sin or virtue, the wrong or right, is judged by those savants by the indication of Divinity from within. Of course receiving Divine signals is not the right of temporal people like us, but it is the privilege of the spiritually advanced. We fail to discern the difference between unethical and trans-ethical. It is because it required that mystic vision and not the incredible brain!

In spiritualism called *adhyātma* also, there is a plethora of enigmatic questions. There are mystics and sages who smoke Ganja (dried leaves of hemp plant) - Why? Why was the great sage Vishwamitra caught under the spell of infatuation? Why was the savant sage of Chandogya Upaniṣad called Raikva seen in an obnoxious, dirty manner, scratching his body and lying under a hand cart? Why did the sage Durvasa have barbaric anger? Why was Lord Krishna described as the pure witness, pure consciousness, free from the three *guṇa-s* despite the fact that he had 16,108 wives? No science can answer these questions satisfactorily, nor can intelligence. But mysticism can answer these questions and obliterate all doubts at once.

The mystic vision is graced by the indwelling Lord. If a seeker in the path of spiritualism treads the path without the grace and without feeling the want of grace, he saddles failure on his back and trudges towards dejection, desperation and sorrow.

Vyasa has said in his commentary on 1/35 of *yoga-sūtra* that even if the smallest bit of mystical experience is had, the whole enigma in metaphysics, religion and spiritualism can pose no threat.

Even if one gets the vision of that which is in the realm of mysticism, it cannot be transmitted, it cannot be theorised, and it cannot be articulated. No polemical skill can come to convince the seeker. Therefore, the most scrupulously precise books of knowledge have articulated those realities with grim silence. One can say by words that sugar is sweet, but the sweetness of sugar cannot be explained or described by even the king amongst poets Kalidasa!

Yoga-system being a *Darśana*, is replete with mystical issues since all metaphysics is mystical. The philosophical mysticism can be traced in its cosmology where the Divinity is kept out of cosmology in the explicit theorisation. But in its implicit dictum, the Divinity has an 'all in all' place. The psychology of yoga clearly holds that the *sattva* is admissible but the *raja* and *tama* are not. Teleology spells out the reality that nothing is totally discardable nor totally admissible in ultimate analysis. The third chapter speaks of all those incredible discernments and powers.

Finally the system yoga streamlines a comprehensive ethico-religious system to develop the capacity and qualify for intuitive mysticism. It defines this faculty as the gateway for spiritual summum bonum. This speaks of the important part of intuitive mysticism in spiritualism and the place of yoga in spiritualism; this tradition has spelt it out so very comprehensively.

❑❑❑

14. YOGA - A *Kalpataru*

Yoga is comparable to the celestial tree called as '*Kalpataru*'. This tree is a wonderful miracle of the heavens; sit under it, make a wish and it is fulfilled in almost no time. Here yoga is compared to this tree not because yoga works so miraculously; but because yoga philosophy, the science of yoga and practical aspects of yoga fulfil all that a human being cherishes. It is a complete and comprehensive system to serve the entire of human being.

The human desires and yearnings are structured on his wants and needs. The social and economic needs of man change depending upon time and place. But some wants and desires have remained unchanged. From the earliest times till this day, neither have these changed nor have these been replaced or displaced. These changeless and perennial desires, yearnings and wants have proved to be universal. No culture, no civilisation, no religion and no socio-economic system has been able to alter or sublate these. No system has ever transgressed, surpassed or obliterated these basic desires, yearnings and wants. These desires are accepted here as basic and universal.

There are two classes of such basic desires. One set comprises of objective wants. These are well known through the social and economic sciences. These are food, clothing and shelter. Of course since these wants are well known and are matter of investigation for socio-economic sciences, we shall not go into investigation of these. Besides, for our purpose it is not essential to do so.

We are going to examine the second set of universal needs which are wholly subjective and 'soul-based'. They do not at all stand ejected even for temporal, materialistic and atheistic people. They are 'soul-based' in the sense that they are woven around the spiritual entity that resides in all human beings.

The needs give rise to desire. Even if the needs are objective, the desires are subjective. This is a psychological fact. Therefore, if the universal subjectivistic desires are projected in the minds of the readers, these can be understood, which we are going to explore and define. Let us now understand what these universal, eternal desires and needs are.

There is no normal human being who would desire to be weak, fragile, or in mental or physical ill-health. As a matter of fact, every one yearns for good health, vitality and vigour. Therefore the first and foremost universal and eternal desire and need is physical and mental health.

Similarly, no normal person desires to be a stupid, ignorant and block-headed imbecile. As a matter of fact, everyone longs to be knowledgeable, wise or even omniscient. Therefore knowledge, scholarship and wisdom are the second universal, eternal desires of human beings.

Likewise no normal human being would like to be in a condition of turmoil, mental agitation, agony, distress and discontent. In other words, everyone yearns for peace, tranquility and contentment. Therefore the three basic spiritual needs, as examined above are :

1) Physical-mental health, strength and vitality

2) Scholarship, wisdom and omniscience

3) Inner peace, tranquility and contentment

Since this triad of human desires, when fulfilled, give the man satisfaction of having fulfilled the purpose of existence and since yoga has the possibility of serving these needs, it has been compared to the wonderful tree of heaven, called *Kalpataru*'.

A society may be in a primitive tribal stage of culture, or socio-economically and technologically advanced and in an affluent stage of civilisation or purely materialistic or highly evolved spiritually. The above needs stand unaltered and undislodged.

The unquenchable universal desire for physical and mental well-being gives rise to the various sciences or branches of knowledge and arts. These are the health sciences ranging from sciences of physical exercises to physiology, hygiene and medicine. These sciences attempt to quench the thirst of desire for health, strength and vitality.

Human endeavour and worship of knowledge and wisdom is just incredibly marvellous. Man has created a plethora of sciences around him to quench his thirst for knowledge. These are natural sciences, physical sciences, psychological sciences, social sciences, speculative sciences, theoretical sciences, normative sciences, prescriptive sciences, and moral ethical sciences.

While for inner peace, tranquility and contentment, there are religious sciences, sciences of meditation, worship sciences

(*Upāsanā Śāstra*) etc. Broadly speaking, we can make a functional classification of all the sciences which serve the three basic human needs:

1) For health- Health sciences (*Ārogya Svāsthya Śāstra*)

2) For knowledge - Scholarship sciences/ eruditory sciences (*Vidyā Śāstra*)

3) For peace -Worship sciences (*Upāsanā Śāstra*)

A human being can experience a sense of accomplishment in life if all the three sets of sciences can satisfy him. When yoga is compared with *Kalpataru*, it is with a factual view that as a science, philosophy and religion, it serves all the three ends to the highest degree.

The wisdom bank or treasury of wisdom has had deposits from time immemorial. These deposits were made by various sciences, philosophies and religions. But it is not an exaggeration to state that yoga as a science, art, philosophy and religion has served that bank, and through it humanity at large more than all the other sciences, philosophies and religions put together, for human upliftment and evolution.

Now we shall analyse the human aspects around which these desires and needs are centred. We will also analyse how yoga serves each of the human components, which will establish the greatness of yoga.

A human being is made up of five aspects and all his wants and desires have their centre in these five aspects. These five aspects of a human being are:

1) Physics of man: This comprises of anatomy and physiology of man. It is constituted by skin, flesh, blood, fat, marrow, bones, muscles and all organs.

2) Psycho physical: This comprises of brain and psycho-sensory and psycho motor system. The contemporaneous activity of body and brain are in the eternal mind, the meta-psyche, whereby the evolution process can be carried over to one's next life and all subsequent lives.

By training the psycho-physics of man, yoga increases intellectual capacities, thereby enabling him through the development of his intellectual faculty to quench his thirst of wisdom.

The inner peace, quietude and tranquility depend upon skill and artistry with which one leads one's life. The relation between art and mental peace needs no explanation. Of course the joy, peace and quietude that come through the ethico-religious and psychological practices of yoga, are beyond the psycho-sensory pleasures. A *yogī* reaps the highest reward by unearthing the deep and rich mine of Spirit and Divinity, which is the central force in all atomic and sub-atomic particles, which constitute the Universe. It is also the central force of a human being. This incalculable glory within, amounts to infinite contentment, peace and satiety. All the desires, passions, and yearnings get obliterated by this supreme realisation. When the Universal Principle is realised within a human being, can ecstasy be measured?

3) Psychics of man: This aspect of man is made up of empirical mind, empirical ego and empirical intelligence called as 'psyche'.

4) Meta-psychics of man: This component is the subtle body or astral body which is subjected to transmigration and accounts for natural dispositions and capacities of a human being since birth.

5) Meta-physics of Man: The Spiritual and Divine entity in man which is Infinite, Immutable and Eternal.

There are no other aspects in a human being besides these five aspects. Yoga, as an art, science, philosophy and religion works on each of these five aspects very circumspectly towards the satisfaction of these basic needs.

Any defect in the physics, psycho-physics and psychics of man gives rise to physical as well as mental diseases and disorders, with the result that the physical, mental, psychological, emotional and intellectual capacities begin to wane. Yoga can serve the human being, for his cure as well as regeneration and evolution. The ethico-religious practices of yoga are capable of creating a very deep impression and inspire religious ideals.

Yoga is *Kalpataru* in another sense. Just as man looks for God's grace in anything, be it his need for a penny or emancipation of his soul, likewise he turns to yoga for all his needs and longings. And just as God does not feel offended for what man seeks from Him, yoga too does not feel offended for what man seeks from it. Today, one takes recourse to yoga for pain, be it a sprained ankle or a psychotic knot in the brain. It is through yoga that the crippled and the feeble have become hale and hearty. The grief-stricken and sorrowful have become joyous and happy. The weak and sickly have become vigorous and healthy. The brutes and savages have become benign and humane. The sensual and carnal have become temperate and abstemious. The impotent and resigned have become potent and retentive. The gluttonous and voracious have become moderate and sober. The temporal and mundane have become ethereal and spiritual. The list can be endless.

Coming to the intellectual urge of man, particularly today when man has grown to be more progressive minded, analytical minded and scientific minded, and also an astute pragmatic and fastidious observer he will surely find that this ancient wisdom richly studded in yoga philosophy does not dabble in anything that can be termed as antiquated or loose thinking. Rather, as a system of philosophy it is sumptuous food for human intelligence and a challenge to human intelligence. Yoga as a system of thought has neither ridiculed logical positivism and intellectual rationalism nor has it belittled the importance of positive sciences. As a matter of fact, it has applied those in its scholastics. Sciences like logic, physics and psychology which are in the forefront today, have not been treated with disdain or rancour, but have been accorded an honoured place in its theories and dialectics. Yoga philosophy has used them as a launching pad to soar upwards towards a complete science. The philosophy of yoga system, with intellectual analysis, impeccable imaginations for hypothesis and pedantics has progressed into the realm of metaphysics to spell out the branches of metaphysics i.e. cosmology, ontology, teleology, and theology.

All these delineations of yoga in the above mentioned branches of metaphysics have been scrupulously analytical, logical and scientific with impeccable theories. The balance that it has struck between logic and abstruse mysticism is just marvellous and astonishing.

Despite the fact that these various branches of metaphysics demand high and rigorous scholasticism, the yoga system unlike the other philosophies has not given undue importance to hair splitting arguments. It has not made this system a battlefield of polemics. The seeds of exceptionally rich scholastics are sown in a relishing proportion. The seeds of metaphysics are sown in the womb of words of the aphorism. Therefore a casual glance through the text of yoga philosophy does not reveal the metaphysical import of these aphorisms. To discern the underlying purport and scholarly treatment of the subject requires a very keen and sharp intelligence. At this point it is needless to say, how yoga system comes to quench the thirst of human intelligence.

One who has the faculty developed for mysticism and one who has the potential for a mystic and poetic vision of life, finds an ocean of most enchanting material. Nevertheless, one who has an alert eye to detect realism finds that his eyes are opened further. And with capacity for higher psychological practices of yoga he reaches the glory that is deep down in the heart and deep under the psyche; automatically closing the eyes out of ecstasy to envision the closed eye perceptions. The realistic intellectualism and abstruse mysticism have perfectly cohesive mingling here.

Finally, tracing the development of peace, quietude and contentment, through yoga, it is needless to point out that it bestows all that which depends upon perfect physical health and mental health. Besides, by satiety to intellectual, emotional, religious and spiritual appetite, yoga stands out amongst all other sciences, arts, philosophies and religions with a distinction. A man who desires religious experiences gets a sumptuous and relishing, bio-electrical and psycho-electrical jolts and tremors of ecstasy, that give boundless and immeasurable, joy, bliss and beatitude.

Now we shall analyse and ascertain how the ethico religious aspects of yoga or the practical aspect of yoga called as '*Aṣṭāṅga yoga*' help towards fulfilling the three soul based and Universal needs of a human being viz.

1) Health,

2) Knowledge and Wisdom,

3) Peace and Contentment.

'*Yama*' and '*Niyama*' make a human being more moderate in his habits and cure all the diseases and troubles that arise on account of intemperance, over-indulgence, immorality and various forms of unethical behaviour. Since the practice of *yama-niyama* principles clear the mind and intelligence, of obscuring *tamas*, the intellectual and emotional fidelity in response to reality is heightened and knowledge is heaped up. Since the two principles make a human being a confirmed moralist, ethical-minded, religious-minded, virgin and spotless, he is caught up in a joyous deluge of peace and contentment.

Āsana is the third aspect of *Aṣṭāṅga yoga*. This is a branch of *Kalpataru* within easy reach of any ordinary aspirant. Even the most worldly individuals find good, robust health, and vitality through practice of *āsana*. There is nothing totally wrong in such materialistic motive. The wise sages of *Vedas* prayed for health, for their unobstructed and unimpeded journey towards God. One may refer to Vedic peace invocation: "Om, let my limbs and speech, *prāṇa*, eyes, ears, vitality and all senses grow in strength" (*Chandogya śānti*) ----" Om, while praising Gods with steady and strong limbs, may we enjoy the life that is beneficial to the gods". (*Muṇḍaka śānti*). Therefore, from materialistic people to spiritual and religious sages, all without exception have expressed a desire for physical and mental well being. No normal person ever desires, or wishfully allows a revolt of the body or its incapacity and debility. The *asana-s* now have a popular position in the advent of health consciousness in people. It has been proved that *āsana-s* do what is required for augmentation of good health in the body-mind system of a human being. The body can be made to subserve the purpose of life with harmony and co-operation as against its baneful protests and revolt against any pursuit of human endeavour that a human being may cherish.

Besides, *āsana-s* have won acclaim for their great capacity to work as an incredible therapy against human suffering.

But religious role of *āsana* characteristic, when practised as an integral part of *Aṣṭāṅga yoga* has a drive and complement towards the bed-rock principle of yoga, 'the mental restraint'. Since the essential yoga has the highest capacity to fulfil the basic spiritual needs of human beings, it will be more appropriate to evaluate the role of *āsana* from that perspective.

To conceive mental restraint without physical and sensory-motor restraint is absurdity itself. Physiologically, one must understand that the mental restraint demands and requires physiological passivity by prevention of impulsiveness of sensory cortex and motor cortex of the brain. Without any inhibition in these two cortices, the nervous system behind sensory organism and the glands that stimulate the inner organism, the restraint that yoga speaks of is an impossibility. The *prāṇa* does that pacification by compending itself. This physiological and cortical pacification and the resultant psycho-sensory and physical pacification take the aspirant away from the bustle, confusion and travail of 'business of life' and bestow the bliss within.

The capacity to effect control over physical, psychosensory and cerebro-cortical fronts, depends upon the freedom in the flow of bio- energy in the human system. The *āsana* helps open out this freedom. The *Yogāsana* helps one develop the capacity to expand and contract, diffuse and convoke the vital energy and to withstand the diffused or convoked state of energy in any part of the physique, physiology and neurology. Through the *āsana* the system can withstand the extraordinary inhibition, hypoactivity and starvation that is effected by *yogīc* restraint. The steadiness that is required in higher practices of yoga from physique to deep physiology is bestowed by *āsana* if done with proper application. We might conclude with a statement that *āsana* has a vital role to play at any stage of human evolution and endeavor, from materialism to the highest spiritualism.

Prāṇāyāma is the fourth aspect of *Aṣṭāṅga yoga*. This too is practised in two ways i.e. a materialistic approach and a *yogīc* approach. Therefore it serves a worldly man as well as one progressing on the spiritual path. The materialistic and worldly man practises with a shallow and selfish outlook. He may practise with zeal, spirit and earnestness, but uses it to overcome exhaustion and lassitude in body, mind and brain. Thereby he is enabled to serve his mundane objectives. Moreover he uses *prāṇāyāma* to exercise the respiratory organs the lungs, the ribs and the intercostal muscles etc, and effect better respiration, circulation and oxygenation of the body and the brain.

Some of the stunt-men of *Hatha yoga* have an incredible craze for psycho-physical side effects which result from *prāṇāyāma*. They develop a capacity for very prolonged inhalation, retention, and exhalation. No doubt such severe practices enable them to acquire super strength and power. But how do they utilise it? Such intense effort is aimed at worldly gain and power or for some stunts to enchant, amuse and astonish people, and thereby win acclaim and recognition.

Besides, like *āsana*, *prāṇāyāma* too has gained currency as a valuable therapy for the treatment of psycho-neuro and respiratory-circulatory disorders.

Let us now highlight the essential role of *prāṇāyāma*. Defining *prāṇāyāma* as breath control is like describing an elephant by its thin and small tail. Such an interpretation and mistaken notion hurts the purist.

Prāṇāyāma is cosmic poetry. *Prāṇa*, according to Indian mystics is a poem of metaphysical reality. *Prāṇa* is the primeval energy and source energy behind all creation in this limitless universe. No manifestation whatsoever is un-*prāṇic*. It is this divine cosmic force that holds together and sustains all manifestations. Besides, this *prāṇa* is the power of the Divinity through which the Divinity fulfils its role as Creator, Sustainer and Absorber or Dissolver of all manifestations. It is *prāṇa* that links the creation with its Creator and the Creator with its Creation. *Prāṇāyāma* is playing the music of macrocosm within the microcosm. It is reflection of macrocosmic reality in the microcosm. Therefore, it is the highest form of prayer, the highest form of worship and the highest form of *yajña* to the Divinity. *Prāṇāyāma* is the process to cosmicalise every corpuscular particle in a human being, and every bit of human blood. Of course this is the essential, metaphysical, cosmic and religious purpose of *prāṇāyāma*. The words are not sufficient to describe it.

But as far as the physics, psycho-physics and psychics of *prāṇāyāma* are concerned, it may be concluded that it enhances the functioning of cerebro-cortical parts of the brain, the cerebro-spinal system, and therefore entire physical psychological, psycho-sensory and psycho-neuro system of human being thereby leading towards *yogīc* restraint of the mind.

Pratyāhāra, dhāraṇa, dhyāna and *samādhi* are the higher aspects of *Aṣṭāṅga yoga*. Unfortunately they too have been exploited and made to wear the garb of spiritualism and Godhood thereby exploiting the masses, because it is more convenient for exploitation through spiritual semblance in these higher aspects of yoga. But we shall waste no more time and space to delineate upon this filthy and foul aspect here.

For a sincere neophyte, meditation or *dhyāna* as it is generally called may be practised, although not on the scrupulous lines of yoga psychology of meditation. Vedic religion and tradition has established the 'Puja-room' meditation, and recitation of hymns based on the compositions of mystic poets and saints. Meditation on the deity of one's liking or *japa* may be done for a few minutes every day which really elevates the worshipper. Ten or fifteen minutes of such religious practices called meditation carry him through the bustle of life with far less tension and fear of persecution. Moreover, man carries out the business of life from a higher pedestal. It is on account of this elated conduct of life of an ardent Hindu, that the conduct of life has stood out in sharp focus from amongst the behaviour of all other communities. The subterranean flow of Hindu Philosophy is a live current in the Hindu way of life.

Let yoga be practised for physical and mundane and forhigher spiritual and religious end, it is not offended even if the aim is not spiritual evolution, but the pursuits must be faithful and honest. After all, a man can draw from this ocean according to his capacity and grace of God.

Since yoga has been compared with *Kalpataru*, there is a dark side to its magnanimity. As a wayfarer on the path of yoga, one cannot refrain from saying that on account of the vast popularity that yoga has gained in our times, some aspects of yoga are being thrust indiscriminately with a spirit of missionarism. This has become a redoubtable endeavour. The vicious people can be at the receiving end for super power and strength, only to become more robust in the abuses of life for yoga fortifies the physical, mental and nervine strength. Just as a devilish brute during sleep, has merely a stop-gap or cessation of his vandal activities that are substantial within him, and just as the brute wakes up with even greater vitality for evil thereafter, the non-integral practices of *āsana*, *prāṇāyāma* and modern meditative techniques by a carnal and hedonist would work as a mere temporary cessation of usual base activities and then erupt with greater force. *Yogīc* pills are swallowed like drugs without dietary regimen of *yama* and *niyama*. It is on this account that yoga may well rove to be more a danger than a boon in the ultimate analysis. The law that "devil must first be weakened before reformation begins", assumes even greater significance and importance in yoga as far as the imparting and spreading of yoga is concerned. Otherwise physical, mental and nervine reinforcement may make an unscrupulous and licentious practitioner even more uncontrollable and unscrupulous and in fact, a danger to society.

❑❑❑

15. The Refutation of Yoga System in Brahmasutra

The refutation of the yoga system that occurs in the *Brahmasūtra* is the most disconcerting matter for the ardent student of yoga philosophy. The fact that the *Brahmasūtra* codifies the *Vedānta-Darśana*, the philosophical system typified by the Vedas and *Upaniṣad*s, cannot be a disposable opponent or a trivial wrangling of the opponent.

Secondly, the yoga-tradition holds Veda-Vyasa, the most faithful and the only commentator on *yoga-sūtra*, as the aphorist of the *Brahmasūtra*. This complicates the engima further and puts the student of yoga philosophy in a most unexplicating dilemma. It becomes inconceivable that the *Brahmasūtra* stand in refutation of the *yogasūtra-s* particularly when the commentator and the aphorist of the two systems is one and the same person.

Moreover any counter argument to the refutation worded in the *Brahmasūtra* becomes nothing different than biting one's own tongue since, it is Vyasa, who is revered as much as Patanjali to the yoga clan, who pens the refutation of the yoga, in the *Brahmasūtra*.

It is truly a greatly disconcerting thing for the Patanjalas since there can be no counter attack mounted or defence propelled because either of the two would mean presenting dialectic and scholastics against the undepreciable, unquestionable and most revered Upanishads.

Therefore, there are some run-away excuses and escapes in the commentaries on the *Brahmasūtra*, arguing that the yoga refuted in the *Brahmasūtra* is not Patanjali's yoga, but something that has since disappeared from the surface of the earth. This stand is not a truly convincing one, because the *Brahmasūtra* has refuted and grounded many other systems with vindictiveness and with a sense of despise. Those philosophies have not lost their trace in total. Therefore on what account it is to be believed that a comparatively minor stroke or punch has resulted into a total defacement of a non-Patanjali yoga system with absolutely no relics left behind. The run-away interpreters have failed in proving the existence of any such non-Patanjalic system of yoga which can substantiate their stand.

What is attempted here is to present a hypothesis that *Brahmasūtra* has refuted Patanjali's *Yoga Darśana*, but on a technical aspect without spirit of staunch opposition.

First of all, it is to be seen where, how and why the *Brahmasūtra* has refuted the *Yoga Darśana*. The second chapter of *Brahmasūtra* is called as 'Avirodha Adhyaya' that separates *smṛti*s which oppose the Vedantic doctrine. There occurs an Adhikarana (a topic) as held by Shankara and Ramanuja and others as 'Yoga Pratyukta Adhikarana'.

The *sūtra* that refutes the yoga philosophy is *etena yogaḥ pratyuktaḥ*– meaning "Therefore yoga too, stands refuted".

Wherefore refuted? The Saṁkhya Smṛti of Kapila is refuted because it holds that the *prakṛti* is an independent material cause of the Universe. If the atheistic Kapila Smṛti is held valid, the theistic text would be with validity sublated, which hold God as the source of the Universe.

The Seshwara Saṁkhya crystallised in Patanjali *Yoga Darśana* also holds that the Universe is produced by the intrinsic potency (Ksetra Śakti) of *prakṛti*. Just as grass and vegetation are produced from the earth duly favoured by rains, the *Mahat* (cosmic principle of intelligence) also serves as a sprout hole for the Universe, with the favour of the God. The Seshwara Saṁkhya, as against the other school of Saṁkhya at least brings God as a contributory factor, while the *prakṛti* is assigned the more prominent and vital role in the cosmological unfoldment. In the eyes of the *Vedānta*, though yoga has admitted Ishwara, it is just ostensible because God is reduced to the status of mere auxiliary force or a contributory factor, in the drawing out what is contained in the womb of *prakṛti*, which is power to germinate and evolve. This power is supposed to be intrinsic to it and in no way developed, and sustained or made ontologically dependent on the Ishwara or the Brahman. The *Brahmasūtra* on the other hand, explicitly declare, at the very beginning of the text;

Janmādiyasyayadaḥ ~ (B.S. 1/1/2)

meaning : "He, from whom proceed the Creation, Preservation and Absorption of the Universe, is Brahman."

Therefore, the position of theistic *Sāṁkhya* falls very much below the expectations of the profused theism of *Brahmasutra*, where God has to be all and not just an auxiliary and contributory factor and titular entity.

The refutation of yoga therefore occurs, not for the difference in metaphysics of yoga or the cosmological processes postulated by yoga or psychology of yoga. But the refutation is on account of non-mention of Ishwara at the helm of the cosmological evolution. It really pricks and wounds the profuse deism of *Brahmasūtra* that the *yoga sūtra* does not make an explicit statement to the effect that *Ishwara* is the whole and sole of Universe. If it had placed the *Ishwara* at the helm of *prakṛti* and not the *prakṛti* at the helm of cosmos, the two systems would have been in complete harmony.

At this point it is to be understood that, the refutation of yoga in the *Brahmasutra* occurs for no other reason or difference of opinion but the only reason that *Ishwara* of the yoga system is more neutral and above the Universal phenomenalism. However the Vedantic Highest entity is the transcendent and immanent principle as explicitly held by the *Brahmasutra*. The profuse deism of *Vedānta* holds that every particle infinitesimally small to infinitely infinite throbs with the Divinity. But the theistic *Sāṁkhya* of Patanjalas find it sufficient to confer, mere flawlessness and faultlessness and unexceedable and inequitable power to the *Ishwara*, in its doctrine. In the view of *Vedānta*, the Patanjalas shirk from admitting the "all in all status" of Brahman. The Patanjalas in their opinion hesitate for some reason or reservations, and avoid any explicit declaration of status of the Divinity as clearly held by the *Brahmasutra*.

The obvious question here is why the *yoga-sūtra* has not boldly declared that the universe ensues from the Lord of Lords, the Divinity, and nature is intrinsically of the nature of the Divinity.

It is true that what *yoga-sūtra* has apparently expressed is the presidency of *Ishwara* over Creation and not premiership over Creation, which has been conferred to the *prakṛti*. One recalls here the quotations from the Bhagawad Gita:

etadyonīni bhūtāni sarvāṇityupadhārayaḥ

ahaṁ kṛtsnasya jagataḥ prabhavaḥ pralayastathā (B.G. VII-6)

"Know that all beings have their birth in this *prakṛti.* I am the source of all this world and its dissolution also". This stanza of the Gita faintly declares that the womb of Creation is *prakṛti* and the Lord is the origin or the president over the cosmological process.

The following stanza :

māyādhyākṣeṇa prakṛtiḥ sūyate sacārācaram I

hetunānena kaunteya jagadviparivartate II (B.G. IX.10)

clearly states "Under my presidency, nature gives birth to all things, sentient and insentient. It is by the *prakṛti* that the world (Universe) revolves". In the fourteenth chapter of the Gita, it is said :

mamayonirmahadbahma tasmin garbham dadhāmyaham I (B.G. XIV.3)

"The great Brahman (*prakṛti*) is my womb, in that I cast the seed (and from that, the birth of beings)". It should be noted in the above stanza that the Lord says "I cast the seed" and not "I am the seed"; and that the womb (the *prakṛti*) stands as material cause of the Universe. The *Ishwara* becomes the springboard for *prakṛti* in so far as He is the President of the Universe.

Now the question, why the *yoga-sūtra-s* do not amplify the reality that *Ishwara* is at the helm of Creation, Sustenance and Dissolution, which is not a trivial fact to be overlooked, denied or repudiated and abnegated, because reality remains to be reality.

Therefore, the master mind of the aphorist makes the position of the doctrine clear that the premiership over Creation etc. lies with *prakṛti* and the presidency with the *Ishwara* . Let us try to reach our hands to the true purport in the *yoga-sūtra*.

The section of *yoga-sūtra* that deals with the *Ishwara* (1/24 - 1/28) clearly states, that *Ishwara* is the *Puruṣa Viśesa*. The very term ' *puruṣa*' vibrates with etymological meaning :

puram śarīram tāsmin śete iti puruṣaḥ I

Meaning: the *puruṣa* is the principle that reposes or is embedded in all embodiments. Therefore His rulership extends over *prakṛti* too. The term *Ishwara* denotes the unexceedable power, splendour, grandeur, glory and magnificence. Therefore it must be understood that the *Ishwara* of the Patanjalas is as much a transcendental principle as is immanent in all the embodiments, be they gross material, supra material, or even trans material.

Secondly with the mention that the '*āuṁ*' connotes Ishwars, there can be no different opinion that *Ishwara* of Patanjala is none other than Brahman of Upanishads and the *Brahmasūtra*.

The *yoga-sūtra-s* do not explicitly mention that *Ishwara* is the womb of Creation and that all the nature is of the nature of Divinity because it goes against the yoga-psychology in its practical aspect. Holding that all material mutations are of the nature of Divinity, the *vairagya* from anything would mean a withdrawal from Divinity. What can be relinquished, if everything and anything in all forms, is divinity? Where comes the question of mental restraint when all the mental modifications pertain to matter, infra-matter, supra-matter and trans-matter, which are of the nature of Divinity? Therefore, no mental rambling would amount to mental digression. Therefore, the Patanjalas distinctly hold *prakṛti* separate from *puruṣa* and *Ishwara* .

Even in the intuitive-mysticism held by yoga and Vedantis, God is to be first revealed in one's own self. This vision is not had outside unless it is had inside. The search for Divinity is inside one's self in a *yogī's* meditation, and in the meditation mentioned in the *Brahma-vidyā* of the Upanishads.

The express mention that Creation ensues from Divinity, would resist the theistic *yogī* to retire from *prakṛti*, and therefore the whole science of yoga would be blown to futility, because one can never be a *yogī* without departing from the *prakṛti* by *vairāgya*.

It has to be admitted, however, that what is implicit in the *Yoga Darshana* is not explicit and that has been critically examined by Vyasa in the *Brahmasūtra*. He has pointed out that, what has been implicitly mentioned in the *yoga-sūtra-s* is not made explicit, but what is explicit is different from what is implicit. Therefore, in a dispassionate analysis, it stands out as a defect, and hence is subjected to refutation for another system of thought. Vyasa as the aphorist of the *Brahmasūtra* has critically examined the *Yoga Darśana* and presented a technical analysis. Therefore, the refutation has to be justified in so far as the *yoga-sūtra-s* have not made explicit what is implicit.

But *yoga-sūtra* too should be regarded as faultless in the matter of dispute, because they have avoided the internal contradiction in theory and practice of the doctrine. Not making the fact explicit, but only implicit, that Creation ensues from *Ishwara* , does not go against the practice of *Vairagya*, because with the major dictum that all Creation is Divine and springs forth from Divinity, would rule out the possibility of restraint from the phenomenal world, for a theistic Patanjala. Therefore, the doctrine of Patanjala keeps God away from phenomenal nature.

❑❑❑